Smart Woman's Guide to PMS and Pain-Free Periods.

Linda Woolven, M.H., C.Ac.

WILEY

John Wiley & Sons Canada, Ltd.

Library and Archives Canada Cataloguing in Publication Data

Woolven, Linda
    The smart woman's guide to PMS and pain-free periods / Linda Woolven.

Includes bibliographical references.

ISBN 978-0-470-15379-6

    1. Premenstrual syndrome—Alternative treatment. 2. Menopause—Complications—Alternative treatment. I. Title.

RG161.W65 2008   618.1'72   C2008-907572-X

Production Credits
Cover design: Adrian So
Interior design and typesetting: Tegan Wallace
Printer: Printcrafters

John Wiley & Sons Canada, Ltd.
6045 Freemont Blvd.
Mississauga, Ontario
L5R 4J3

Printed in Canada

1 2 3 4 5 PC 12 11 10 09 08

This book is printed with biodegradable vegetable-based inks. Text pages are printed on 60 lb. Enviro 100 paper, 100% post-consumer waste.

I would like to dedicate this book to women everywhere who want to take back their own power by learning to help, heal and empower themselves. to bring a healthy balance into their lives.

Contents

Acknowledgments

To all the women who helped me over the years to learn more, and want to learn more, in order to help women. To my clients who have inspired me with how effective change, growth and healing can be.

To the many wonderful people writing about women's health: herbalists, naturopaths and other fabulous authors. To those who weren't afraid to share their own experiences and those of their family, clients and friends.

To all the medical doctors who gave me a reason to want to do better and find a healthier solution for women and myself.

I'd like to thank Ted Snider, who helped me to proofread this work and envision it every step of the way. Thanks also to my mom, who has always been down to earth, straightforward and comfortable talking about women's bodily functions and who taught me to be the same. To all my female friends, who could just talk about anything, anytime. To Leah Fairbank who helped make this book into a "must-have" usable guide for women with a clear straightforward message. And to all the people at Wiley who helped make this book a reality.

Introduction

I remember first hearing about periods as a child. There was an aura of mystery about them, and they were spoken of in hushed whispers. I wondered what it was all about. The young women I knew were often not feeling well once a month. At twelve I learned more about this great mystery when I got my first period. It seemed okay at first: I even remember feeling proud. I was changing into a woman and had joined the great mystery. I was capable of bringing about new life.

A few months later, I began to know that not so wonderful feeling many women face: I felt my first period pain. It wasn't severe, and I thought I could easily handle it. Later it became more severe, and I began to get irritable and moody just before it began. Then I got bloated, tired and felt generally poor. I was told that all women go through this, and that I must learn to live with it.

I went to my doctor, and she gave me painkillers. She said women could at least deal with the pain: there was no need to suffer anymore. The painkillers did not deal with my other symptoms. After a while they did not even deal particularly well with the pain. I, like many women, began to try to just live with it, as I had been told to do. I thought that there was no other choice.

If you are like most women, you have probably been told that you just have to endure the discomfort of the monthly cycle. For hundreds of years this is exactly what women have been told. Actually, right up into the 1950s, women were being told that the pain was all in their heads, that it was psychological, that they were hypochondriacs or unable to tolerate normal pain.

Years passed. Then, one day I picked up a book written by a woman herbalist who said that it was not normal for a woman to experience anything more than very mild pain and discomfort with her cycle, if anything at all. At first, I didn't believe it. It was not what I had been told. She claimed the symptoms that preceded and accompanied menstruation were not normal; if a woman had those symptoms her body was out of balance.

The good news is that that herbalist was right. You do not have to suffer the pain of a period—technically called dysmenorrhea—or the many symptoms of premenstrual syndrome (PMS): moodiness, irritability, emotional fragility, acne, bloating, weight gain or water retention, depression, headache, cravings for foods, anxiety, breast pain, backaches, diarrhea or constipation, tension, dizziness, altered sex drive or fatigue. You don't have to suffer period pain caused by a spasming, cramping uterus and poor period flow. Fortunately, there is great relief to be found from all of these symptoms.

Herbs, vitamins, diet and other lifestyle changes can make every day of the month as good as any other day: there need be no pain, no diminished activity and no unpleasant symptoms. And it gets even better: many women report increased creativity around the time of their periods. How is this possible?

That is exactly what this book will help you to discover: healthy, happy, easy cycles, every month, every year, for the rest of your menstruating life. You'll also learn how you can have an easy, symptom-free menopause. We'll look at common health problems related to cycles and hormone balance: premenstrual syndrome (PMS), cramping and pain (dysmenorrhea), lack of periods (amenorrhea) and too much bleeding (menorrhagia). We'll also look at osteoporosis, common pregnancy issues, fibrocystic breast disease, ovarian cysts, uterine fibroids, endometriosis and weight gain. If you create balance in your hormones and your body, you can wipe out every one of these health concerns.

We'll look at the failure of conventional medicine to offer healing solutions to these very real problems. You'll see how diet, vitamins, herbs and supplements can correct the underlying causes.

This book is designed to help women help themselves. It offers easy-to-follow, safe and effective solutions for common health issues. Women can achieve hormonally balanced health fairly quickly by using a natural health approach. Finally, women can remain active and live pain free through their cycles. Even women who have suffered for decades can find relief with a little help from nature.

Sample protocols

Throughout the book, I offer sample case studies and protocols. They provide a clear account of how herbalists, counselors and acupuncturists use herbs, vitamins, nutrition, acupuncture and counseling to treat symptoms and imbalances associated with PMS and other related conditions. The protocols give you an effective place to start. For further guidance, see a natural practitioner. Those on drugs or with serious illnesses are best to see a practitioner to work with them.

1

The Normal Menstrual Cycle

To better understand PMS, painful periods and other menstrual problems, it's a good idea to first understand a healthy menstrual cycle. If you know what your body is doing, you start to take control of it and work with it to bring about healthy changes.

For the most part, your monthly cycle is controlled by two areas of your brain—the hypothalamus and the pituitary gland—and by your ovaries. Every month, your body secretes hormones that ensure your ovaries release only one egg. These same hormones also get the lining of your uterus ready to house the egg. This cycle is instigated by a change in the two most important female sex hormones: estrogen and progesterone.

The hypothalamus is in charge of your female hormonal system. It releases hormones that in turn encourage your pituitary gland to release follicle-stimulating hormone (FSH) and luteinizing hormone (LH).

During the first stage of the menstrual cycle, FSH helps mature the egg by producing estrogen. When the levels of estrogen get high enough, your pituitary gland stops producing FSH and starts producing LH. The main job of LH is to start ovulation, the release of the egg. When estrogen and LH are both at their peak, the egg is released from its neat little sac—called a follicle—in the ovaries into the fallopian tube, which connects the ovaries with the uterus. Once in the uterus, the egg starts its journey toward possible fertilization: pregnancy.

The empty ovarian follicle is now called the corpus luteum. Its main job is to make progesterone, which helps ensure that the fertilized egg is well housed in the uterine lining. It is here that the baby grows in the uterus should the egg become fertilized.

If the egg is not fertilized, you are not pregnant, your progesterone production goes down and your period begins about two weeks later. Then the cycle begins again, and continues until you become pregnant or reach menopause.

When all this is functioning normally—when your hormones and nutrients are all properly balanced—you should have a pain-free (or virtually pain-free) cycle, with no mood changes and no uncomfortable PMS symptoms.

The normal menstrual cycle takes about twenty-eight days to complete. Some women's cycles are a few days less and some are more, so don't worry if yours is not exact. As long as you're not getting any symptoms and your cycle is within four to five days of the typical twenty-eight-day cycle, it is normal.

The cycle is divided into three distinct phases: follicular, ovulatory and luteal. The follicular lasts for ten to fourteen days; the ovulatory, the shortest phase, for about thirty-six hours; and the luteal for about fourteen days.

Unfortunately, many women—most of us—do not have a so-called normal cycle, and we suffer from various problems, such as premenstrual syndrome (PMS), painful periods (dysmenorrhea), heavy periods (menorrhagia), lack of periods (amenorrhea), breast or ovarian cysts, fibroids, endometriosis, weight gain, common pregnancy and menopause issues. There are important links between your menstrual cycle and the development of osteoporosis.

Let's take a closer look at these issues and learn how to correct them.

2

Understanding PMS

At one time, people believed PMS was all in a woman's head and doctors prescribed antidepressants and other drugs. Now PMS is slowly being recognized as a serious, growing issue for women. Between 30 and 40 percent of women suffer from PMS; 10 percent are severely incapacitated for part of the month.[1] These figures are probably low, since many women do not seek help for PMS.

Clinically, I would say that this statistic should be much higher. Almost every woman I see, even if she comes in for other health concerns, has some imbalances in her cycle. PMS seems to strike women in their thirties and forties, although certainly younger and older women suffer from it.

Many physicians still don't recognize PMS, even though it was clinically defined more than sixty years ago. And so, conventional medical practitioners rarely give PMS sufferers the help they need. Instead they give drugs for depression (Prozac and Zoloft) or for anxiety (Valium), or they prescribe hormones. This situation makes a hard choice for women—as, of course, all women want relief from the pain and discomfort of PMS, but they may not know that there are other drug-free choices that offer real solutions without the side effects and unnecessary risks of the drugs. So they take the recommended drugs, many of which are risky, and they experience side effects. Some drugs may help with the symptoms, but often they don't treat the underlying imbalances in the body. Fortunately, natural herbs and vitamins can help balance the body, eliminate unpleasant symptoms and make the body healthier—all without side effects or risks.

Some doctors treat the symptoms of premenstrual syndrome by putting women on the birth control pill or Anaprox, an anti-inflammatory painkiller. I took Anaprox for years, and though it masked my discomfort for several months, it also caused a serious side effect: an ulcer. Both drugs can pose significant risks, once again forcing a woman to make hard choices, especially when she may feel that she has no choice. I certainly was told of no other choice at my doctor's office. Many women believe there is no alternative to prescription drugs. And the drugs don't offer help at the fundamental level: they don't treat all of the causes of premenstrual syndrome.

Drug Risks

Just what are the risks of these drugs? Anti-inflammatory drugs, such as aspirin and Anaprox, can cause stomach and intestinal ulcers, bleeding and wear on the digestive system, they can also diminish the cartilage in joints A hard choice: a risk of ulcers and arthritis, or period pain and PMS?

Aspirin and Tylenol (acetaminophen) are often given for period pain. Both are toxic to the liver and kidneys. If you take Tylenol at the maximum recommended daily dose even for a short time, you stress your liver.[2] Both Aspirin and Tylenol suppress the immune system.

The Pill can reduce some of the symptoms of PMS and other hormone-related symptoms, but like other drugs, it carries risks. The biggest risks are that it is linked with heart disease, stroke, and even some cancers, and many women find they can't get pregnant for a long time after coming off the pill. It also reduces certain key nutrients in the body; lack of those nutrients can cause PMS (see Chapter 4 for a full discussion). Even if you choose to stay on the pill, there are many herbs and supplements you can safely take with the pill to correct underlying hormone-related issues and make your cycle a healthier one.

Exactly What Is PMS?

PMS is a condition that reoccurs at the time of ovulation, a few days to fourteen days before menstruation. More than 150 symptoms have been attributed to premenstrual syndrome, including depression; fatigue; irritability; anxiety; headaches; mood swings; altered sex drive; altered eating habits and cravings for food like salt, sugar and fat; acne; backache; bloating; water retention; weight gain; diarrhea; constipation; tension; altered moods; dizziness; uterine cramps (although this is more a symptom of dysmenorrhea); abdominal and breast pain, tenderness and distention.

There is help for PMS from natural medicine, which seeks to correct the underlying causes of PMS and adjust them, using diet, herbs, vitamins and other supplements. Many women can find complete relief from PMS using a combination of these factors, even after being told for years by conventional medicine that they just have to live with it, or after being given painkillers that never addressed the underlying problems and did nothing to cure the illness.

As a master herbalist, counselor and acupuncturist—who uses the full realm of herbs, vitamins, supplements and nutrition—I have seen women with extreme PMS (who were so depressed they were having suicidal thoughts) go on to make a full recovery by following a natural health regimen of herbs, vitamins, minerals and lifestyle and nutritional changes.

CHAPTER TWO

One Woman's Case

One woman in particular deserves mention. She came to me extremely depressed, irritable and suffering many of the symptoms of premenstrual syndrome. She was a vegetarian, and in general her diet was pretty good, but she drank large amounts of coffee. And she had a weakness for chocolate. She also had a great deal of stress in her life: she was a single mom raising children by herself and working full-time. She was on the birth control pill.

After an initial assessment, I determined that a combination of herbs and vitamins would be best for her, and I recommended that she slowly reduce (and if possible cut out) her use of caffeine and chocolate. She felt it was not practical to go off the pill, so I recommended supportive therapy. She was given calcium and magnesium, B vitamins with extra B6, a multivitamin-mineral combination and a formula that contained chastetree berry, dandelion root and St. John's wort.

I told her not to expect anything for at least three months (sometimes healing takes time), but after one cycle she already felt improvement, and she called to tell me. She sounded like a different women: happier and with hope. After three months, her health began to improve dramatically. She began to return to her optimistic self, she was no longer irritable, anxious or depressed, and she no longer had suicidal thoughts. She stopped gaining weight, her bloating went away, her skin cleared, her period cramping and breast pain greatly diminished, and she had good energy. It is now several years later, and she is doing fantastic. She is still on the pill, so she takes a few maintenance herbs to undo the damage the pill can cause.

I also learned something from her: women who can't or do not want to follow a complete natural health program can still find relief from PMS.

3

The Causes of PMS

A woman's normal menstrual cycle depends on many different factors for it to be regular and without problems. PMS occurs when there is a problem in any one of the intricate reactions between the many organs and glands involved in menstruation.

Although there are a number of factors that can cause PMS, the main cause (that has been found in women with PMS symptoms) is elevated estrogen levels and lowered progesterone levels. Other important causes include:

- Hypothyroidism. An underactive thyroid can cause hormonal problems. Correcting the hypothyroidism often eliminates PMS.
- Elevated levels of the hormone prolactin. Too much prolactin can cause breast tenderness or pain.
- Elevated levels of aldosterone, a hormone produced by the adrenal glands. Too much aldosterone causes sodium retention, which causes water retention, resulting in weight gain and breast tenderness.
- Elevated levels of cortisol. Too much of this adrenal hormone can make you feel anxious, irritable, depressed and emotionally unstable. Stress causes the high cortisol.
- Low progesterone. Failure of the corpus luteum, the empty ovarian follicle, to produce enough progesterone causes a hormonal imbalance.
- Depression.
- Nutritional deficiencies.[1]

You can use natural health remedies to balance your cycle, correct the underlying problems, eradicate PMS—and feel better than you have in years.

Four Types of PMS

Often PMS is divided into different classifications, based on causes and major symptoms.[2] Knowing which classification you fit into can help you to better understand the best way to solve your problem. But don't worry about trying to figure out exactly which classification you fit into: most women fit into several categories. Actually, most of my clients do. Later in the book, in Chapter 6, we will discuss supplements and herbs that will help with your specific symptoms. It is really later in the book, when we look at the supplements and see which one helps with which problem, that the categories and their symptoms become more relevant.

Category 1: caused by high estrogen levels and low levels of progesterone. Its main symptoms are anxiety, irritability, nervous tension and cravings for sweets and carbohydrates. High levels of estrogen can also cause low serotonin, which can lead to depression. This category is the most common.

Category 2: caused by excess amounts of the adrenal hormone aldosterone, which causes your body to retain sodium and water. Common symptoms are edema, bloating, pain in the breasts and weight gain.

Category 3: caused by low magnesium levels in red blood cells and by alterations in the body's regulation of blood sugar. Typical symptoms include cravings for sweets, increased appetite, heart palpitations, fatigue, fainting, headaches and mood swings.

Category 4: caused by low estrogen levels, high progesterone levels. and sometimes elevated androgens in the blood. Symptoms are depression, sleep disturbances, lack of coordination, confusion and loss of concentration; high androgens can cause acne. This category is the least common.

The last three categories will be useful to keep in mind as we go through the different deficiencies and treatments later in the book. But first, let's take a look at the most common category: an elevated ratio of estrogen to progesterone.

Elevated Estrogen

This altered hormone ratio contributes to PMS in many ways. Let's take a closer look at these factors.

Elevated Estrogen Wreaks Havoc on Liver Function

Dr. Morton Biskind developed a theory in the early 1940s that PMS is caused by a decreased ability of the liver to detoxify. A toxic liver causes excess estrogen levels. In a vicious cycle, the buildup of estrogen causes the liver to be even more sluggish so that it puts out less bile and is even less able to get rid of toxins, which leads to even more estrogen in your body and causes PMS.

ONE SIMPLE NUTRIENT YOU CAN TAKE TO HELP THE LIVER DETOXIFY

Probiotics

To help the liver detoxify and return to normal, it is important to establish properly balanced intestinal flora—the normal bacteria that should exist in everyone's digestive system. You can balance your bacteria with probiotics such as acidophilus and bifidus.

---

continued

One of the ways that the liver detoxifies estrogen is to bind glucuronic acid—a naturally occurring substance in your body—to the estrogen, which it then excretes in the bile. But unfriendly intestinal bacteria make an enzyme that breaks the bonds between the glucuronic acid and the estrogen, allowing the estrogen to be released and reabsorbed by the body. Friendly flora fight the unfriendly bacteria, allowing the liver to detoxify excess estrogen.

Elevated Estrogen Increases Pain and Creates Anxiety and Depression

Increased estrogen levels reduce your body's endorphins. Endorphins are responsible for elevating mood and relieving pain; yet women with PMS often have low endorphin levels, so it is not surprising that women with elevated estrogen have more pain, anxiety and depression.[3]

Stress also lowers endorphins. So women who lead stressful, unbalanced lives have more pain and mood imbalances than women whose lives are well balanced. It's important for women to try to reduce stress by exercise, meditation or whatever works. Incidentally, exercise elevates endorphins, improving mood and relieving pain.

Low Serotonin Can Lead to Depression

Increased ratios of estrogen to progesterone reduce your body's serotonin levels. Serotonin is your body's own antidepressant. Most pharmaceutical antidepressants, for example, Prozac, work by making more serotonin available to your brain. Women with PMS have lower levels of serotonin, which explains the depression so common in PMS. If you bring your hormones into balance, your serotonin levels return to normal, and you begin to feel much better.

Conventional doctors treat the depression that comes with PMS by prescribing antidepressants. These drugs do little to alleviate the cause of PMS, but they can—as anyone who takes them knows—cause a host of side effects. Yet more than 80 percent of the twelve million American patients on Prozac are women between twenty-five and fifty years old: the ages at which women are most likely to suffer from PMS.

Fortunately, there are many safe and effective natural remedies that alleviate these symptoms. These remedies—discussed in the upcoming chapters—should be introduced slowly under a herbalist or a natural practitioner's care, allowing women who are on pharmaceuticals to wean slowly off their drugs under supervision. I have done this with scores of women safely and effectively.

There are also many natural, safe and effective remedies to help lower estrogen which will be discussed later.

STRESS AND SEROTONIN

When your body is under stress, your adrenal glands produce more cortisol, which reduces your brain's levels of the amino acid tryptophan. Tryptophan is converted into serotonin, so less tryptophan means less serotonin. Low serotonin is one cause of PMS, and depression is known to make PMS more severe.[4] Prolonged stress can cause your adrenal glands—which help your body deal with stress—to atrophy and become less effective. So, to effectively treat PMS, reduce your stress.

In the chapters to come, you will discover many safe and effective ways to support your adrenal glands and to find a healthy hormonal balance.

Estrogen Goes Up, B6 Goes Down

Elevated estrogen reduces the action of B6, a vitamin that is very important to proper hormone balance and to the manufacture of serotonin. As you now know, lowered levels of serotonin lead to depression and to worse PMS. Supplementing B6 helps this problem while also reducing the excessive estrogen and increasing the deficient progesterone. Birth control pills and estrogen replacements (for example, Premarin) lower levels of vitamin B6,[5] so this advice is especially important to women taking these drugs.

Elevated Estrogen Increases Water Retention

Increased estrogen contributes to PMS in still other ways: it increases aldosterone levels, a hormone produced by the adrenal glands. Too much aldosterone means too much sodium, which causes water retention—a common symptom of PMS.

Elevated Estrogen Increases Breast Pain

Excessive estrogen—produced by your body or taken in the form of the birth control pill—causes prolactin levels to go up. Excess prolactin causes breast pain.

Plastics and chemicals also can increase estrogen levels, so avoid storing food in them as much as possible.

The Thyroid Connection: Another Very Common Cause of PMS

The New England Journal of Medicine published a study that revealed that fifty-one out of fifty-four women with PMS suffered from low thyroid function. In the control group, zero out of twelve women had low thyroid function. When these women were treated for thyroid insufficiency, all PMS symptoms went away. [6] As many as 20 percent of all women suffer from hypothyroidism; many of these cases go undetected.

While conventional medical practitioners use blood tests to diagnose thyroid problems, it is not the only way. Some practitioners also use the basal body temperature test: your body's resting temperature. The test is performed upon awakening on the second, third and fourth day of your period. When you wake up, take your temperature by placing the thermometer under your armpit for ten minutes without moving from your bed. The results should be shown to a natural practitioner so that he or she can help you to determine if you really have an underactive thyroid. Temperatures below 97.8 degrees may mean you do have hypothyroidism. All women with PMS should be screened for thyroid problems.

But don't worry: if you have an underactive thyroid, there are natural ways to help correct it. A properly functioning thyroid means less PMS. See a practitioner to ensure your thyroid is functioning properly, as thyroid levels can change frequently.

4

The Conventional Approach to PMS

There are fabulous, safe and effective natural treatments for each of the many symptoms and underlying causes of PMS: women do not have to suffer PMS silently. By making gradual changes, women will be feeling so good about their cycles, they'll want to share what they've learned with their friends and relatives.

Let's start with what happens to most women when they go to their doctor about their PMS symptoms. In the standard protocol, doctors give women one or more of the following drugs: birth control pills; Prozac or other antidepressant drugs; Valium or other anxiety and insomnia drugs; and Naproxen an aspirin-like painkiller. Some of these drugs can sometimes reduce certain symptoms—but often by masking the symptoms, not by correcting the underlying problem.

Birth Control Pill

Exactly what are the side effects of taking this drug? The birth control pill depletes magnesium, folic acid, vitamins B6, B1, B2, B3 and B12, vitamin C, zinc and manganese.[1,2] Many of these same nutrients are already low in women with PMS, and these same nutrients are used to effectively treat PMS! So, obviously, taking the pill can contribute to the underlying causes of PMS and actually make it worse. The pill can also cause weight gain, depression, headaches, nausea and fluid retention; it can increase levels of cholesterol and triglycerides; it can cause liver disease, urinary tract infections and blood clots; it can deplete folic acid, which can lead to cervical dysplasia.[2,3] Tori Hudson, ND, suggests that it is even linked to certain types of cancers, such as breast and cervical cancers. It can take months, even years, for women who stop taking the pill to have a normal cycle, which makes conception difficult.

Valium

Valium is commonly prescribed for PMS. It's addictive and not designed for long-term use. Its numerous side effects include dizziness, drowsiness, impaired coordination, allergic reactions, headaches, blurred vision, nausea, indigestion, constipation, lethargy, aggressiveness, hallucinations, suicidal feelings, abnormal sleep patterns, confusion, amnesia and depression. People who take Valium wake up with a hangover effect and feel tired. Some people who stop taking Valium experience nightmares, anxiety, irritability, panic, insomnia, nausea, headaches, memory loss, depression, seizures, hallucinations, paranoia and lack of concentration.[4] The drug does not correct any of the underlying causes of PMS or hormonal imbalance.

Naproxen

Naproxen is a nonsteroidal anti-inflammatory drug, like aspirin; it can cause gastrointestinal bleeding, ulcers, iron loss, and irritation of your gastrointestinal tract. Naproxen has also been linked to kidney dysfunction, liver damage, increased blood potassium levels, sodium retention, water retention, bruising, drowsiness, dizziness and blurred vision. Nonsteroidal anti-inflammatory drugs erode the cartilage around the joints and inhibit cartilage repair, which can mean joint damage like arthritis.[5] The drugs do not correct the problems that cause PMS.

Prozac

Prozac, used to relieve depression, belongs to a class of drugs called selective serotonin reuptake inhibitors. It is associated with numerous side effects, including nausea, headaches, anxiety, nervousness, insomnia, drowsiness, diarrhea, dry mouth, loss of appetite, sweating, tremors and rashes. Prozac inhibits sexual function, including loss of libido, and diminishes sexual response. As many as 34 percent of patients report sexual side effects when taking Prozac. [6]

But perhaps the most frightening problem associated with Prozac is that it can lead to violent, destructive outbursts and even suicidal reactions. The number of suicide attempts and deaths that result from people taking Prozac is alarming. There are no long-term studies of people taking Prozac, so we don't know if it's safe. It doesn't correct the hormonal imbalances that cause PMS.

From Drugs to Natural Relief: A Protocol

There is natural relief, even if you have been using drugs to treat PMS for decades. Please note that it is imperative you make the transition from some pharmaceuticals to natural treatments under the care of a qualified practitioner.

A woman, let's call her Sara, came to me after having severe PMS symptoms and painful, heavy periods for more than twenty years. She was on Anaprox for pain and had tried several different antidepressants and was still on one of them. She was feeling desperate. She began a weekly supervised program that would slowly wean her off these drugs and onto herbs. The program included counseling, acupuncture, herbs, vitamins and nutritional changes, all of which we incorporated gradually into her daily routine.

Week 1: *Consultation*
- *Chastetree berry: 225 mg of a standardized tablet a day, to balance hormones*
- *Calcium: 1,200 mg, with food, for cramping*

continued

CHAPTER FOUR

- *Magnesium: 600 mg, with food, for hormone balance and cramping*
- *Cramp bark: 40 drops as needed, up to 4 times per day, to alleviate cramping, empty stomach*

At the end of Week One, Sara stopped taking Anaprox.

Week 2: *Focus on reducing heavy periods and balancing hormones.*
- *First acupuncture session to rebalance hormones and reduce heavy periods*
- *A small amount of 5-HTP for depression and anxiety, while slowly reducing her antidepressant drug, under supervision, a little bit every two weeks*
- *Skullcap and passionflower: 40 drops of each, 3 times per day, on an empty stomach, for anxiety and trouble sleeping*
- *Yarrow: 40 drops, 4 times per day, on an empty stomach, for heavy periods*
- *Liquid iron: 30 mg a day, with food, for blood loss, until blood tests show normal levels*

Sara got her period in Week Two, and for the first time in twenty years she had no pain.

Week 3: *Focus on balancing hormones and reducing depression.*
- *Two acupuncture sessions*
- *Counseling session: how to reduce stress in her life and cope better*

Sara cut out caffeine this week.

Sara started to feel far less stressed.

Week 4: *Focus on reducing depression and weaning off of drugs.*
- *One acupuncture session*
- *One counseling session*
- *B-complex: 50 mg, twice a day, with food, for hormone balance*
- *Increased dosage of 5-HTP*

Week 5:
- *One acupuncture session*
- *One counseling session*

Sara cut out simple sugars from obvious sources and began to eat more fruit, vegetables, whole grains and legumes.

Week 6:
- *One acupuncture session*
- *One counseling session*
- *Increased dosage of 5-HTP and eliminated antidepressants*

Sara felt great. She was no longer depressed or anxious, her periods were lighter, she didn't crave foods before her periods and she was no longer in pain from them. She was amazed and relieved: after years of struggling with these issues without success she had found real help that works.'

Weeks 7 to 10:

☒ *One acupuncture session*
☒ *One counseling session*

Sara was feeling so good by Week Ten that we decided to move to monthly sessions. Her monthly visits were great; we checked in every two months, then as needed.

Years later, Sara is feeling fantastic, and her body is in such good balance that she takes only B-complex, calcium and magnesium daily: she takes the cramp bark every now and again. Her regime keeps her bones strong, her energy good and her body balanced. She no longer gets PMS or any bad symptom related to her period.

In Chapter 5 we take a closer look at natural medicine and easy-to-implement lifestyle changes so you can take control of your monthly cycles and experience pain-free periods!

5

The Natural Approach to PMS: Dietary Changes

L et's begin with some numbers. In a landmark nutritional analysis reported by Guy Abraham, MD, PMS sufferers typically consumed 62 percent more refined carbohydrates than other women, 275 percent more refined sugar, 79 percent more dairy products, 78 percent more sodium, 53 percent less iron, 77 percent less manganese and 52 percent less zinc.[1]

Christiane Northrup, MD, reports that, compared to women who have regular periods, women with PMS consume more animal fat and caffeine from coffee, chocolate and soft drinks and less whole grains and vegetables. These eating habits can lead to increased symptoms of PMS. Women with PMS also have low levels of magnesium and selenium, as well as vitamins C, E and B.

So what can you eat to avoid PMS? We'll look in a bit. But before we do, I want to address an issue that concerns everyone who wants to make changes. I know changes can be challenging, and, for some, dietary changes are especially difficult. Some people like to jump right in and do it all at once, some like gradual changes, and some like to make changes with help from an expert, like an herbalist or another natural health practitioner. Whatever means works for you, go for it: make it as individual as you like. Start as slowly, or quickly, as you need to, and don't be afraid to start small and work your way up. Most people find that as they begin to feel better, the foods they crave change dramatically, and further changes become easier.

As your diet comes to follow this list more and more closely, the changes will be more and more profound: and not just with hormonal balance, but in all areas of your health. You'll feel better than you have in years. And many of the changes are easy: for example, you'll be asked to add *more* foods to your life than you are likely eating right now. Soon you won't have any desire for the old way of life—you'll simply feel too good to go back!

Healthy Diet: In a Nutshell

So what can you eat to avoid PMS? Here's a basic list.

- Increase your consumption of fiber. Fiber is found only in plant-based foods, like whole grains, vegetables, fruit, legumes, sea vegetables, seeds and nuts. Ideally, move toward a vegetarian diet.
- Reduce your consumption of saturated fats.
- Increase your consumption of essential fatty acids.
- Reduce your intake of simple sugars and simple carbohydrates.

- Reduce (and ideally eliminate) caffeine from your diet. This includes coffee, chocolate, regular tea and soft drinks. This may be a hard change to make, so you may want to start slowly. It's a very important change.
- Reduce salt from the diet: this includes table salt, sea salt and soy sauce. Watch for hidden salt, for example, in prepared foods.
- Avoid plastics, pesticides and other chemicals that increase estrogen levels.
- Buy organic produce.
- Avoid packaged foods.
- Make soy foods a regular part of your diet.
- Consume foods rich in sulfur.

What to Eat

It's actually really simple. To ensure a diet that is rich in nutrients, and to prevent and treat PMS and balance hormones, include these wonderful foods in your diet (they will also help prevent all of the other big diseases):

FIGHTING PMS WITH BROCCOLI?

Try to eat as close to a vegetarian diet as you can. The reason for a vegetarian diet is simple: it prevents and treats many major illnesses, including PMS. Almost all vegetarian women eat more fiber and less of the "bad" fats and, as a result, they suffer less from PMS and other estrogen-related diseases like breast cancer. Vegetarians excrete two to three times more estrogen, and have half the free estrogen in their blood than do women who eat meat.[2] Vegetarian women who also watch the other offending foods can do even better. For those who are not vegetarian, don't panic! If you increase the fiber, the plant-based foods in your diet, while reducing the animal products and follow the other suggestions given above, it will take you a long way towards healing and you will feel the results.

Food Categories	Servings Per Day	Examples
WHOLE GRAINS	4 to 9 servings	Choose a wide variety of grains—don't rely on wheat only. Try buckwheat, rye, barley, oats, teff, quinoa, millet, brown rice, etc.
VEGETABLES	6 to 8 servings or more	Include at least one deep leafy green daily like chard, kale, collard greens, broccoli, spinach, beet greens or Chinese greens like bok choy. Yellow, orange, white, purple and red vegetables should also be included frequently.

continued

Food Categories	Servings Per Day	Examples
SPROUTS	Eat freely	Sprouts like broccoli, radish, alfalfa, mung-bean and red-clover are a powerhouse of nutrition. Use them in sandwiches; salads or as a snack.
LEGUMES	1 to 3 servings or more	Soy, lentils, black beans, mung beans, kidney beans, romano beans, pinto beans, chickpeas, etc. Try hummus, soy burgers and dogs, tofu, soy milk, soy ice cream, lentil soups, bean chili, bean soup, Jamaican beans and rice dishes, bean salads, Indian dal, bean dips and Ethiopian wats (bean stews).
NUTS & SEEDS	A handful or more	Include raw unsalted nuts, such as almonds and hazelnuts, and seeds, such as pumpkin, sesame, flax and sunflower. Carry them around for quick and easy snacks.
FRUIT	Minimum of 2 to 3 servings or (preferably) more	Try all of the raw fruits (e.g., apples, grapes, oranges, grapefruit, mangos, kiwi, berries, pomegranate, pears, plums peaches, pineapple, mangosteen, etc.), as well as baked fruits, fruit purees, fruit muffins and fruit cakes—made with whole grain flour and sweetened with fruit—and fruit salads.

Eating Raw

Try to eat many of your vegetables raw: they have better nutritional value and provide the live enzymes you need for digestion. One of the easiest ways to up your raw vegetables is to eat a large salad every day. Also great and easy are delicious fresh juices.

Eating for Variety

Eat a wide variety of foods to prevent both nutritional deficiencies and food allergies.

Eating Fiber

The high-fiber, colorful and nutritious diet listed above lowers estrogen. It partially does this by encouraging friendly flora in the intestines; these flora lower glucuronidase activity (see pages 15–16) and help you eliminate estrogen. Some experts recommend that you eat at least 35 grams (a little less than 1½ ounces) of fiber a day.

Avoiding Allergens

Also avoid suspected food allergens. Food allergies are believed to be one of the possible causes of PMS. Common allergens are wheat, dairy, caffeine, corn, chemical additives, tomatoes, peppers, oranges, shellfish, beef, gluten and soy. Find out what you are allergic to. Two of the best ways to do this are you can go on a food elimination/rotation diet. (This involves cutting all known food allergens out of your diet for at least two weeks and then reintroducing them slowly one at a time, keeping track of any symptoms. It is best to work with a health practitioner on this one.) The other way to find out what you are allergic to is to take the enzyme-linked immunosorbent assay (ELISA) test, which is a blood test done in a lab. ELISA is far superior to the conventional scratch test for detecting food allergies. Once food allergens are out of your life, you'll be surprised by how great you feel.

Increase Good Fats, Reduce Bad Fats

Forget what you have been hearing for years about cutting fat from your diet—you actually need to consume *more* fats. That's right, eat more fat. But *good* fat! Not all fats are created equal: good fats, also called essential fatty acids, actually can improve PMS symptoms and overall health, while bad fats make PMS symptoms worse. Good fats include oils like evening primrose oil, flaxseed oil, borage oil and hemp seed oil. Essential fatty acids (EFAs) are involved in numerous body processes, and they are imperative to overall health. Your body cannot manufacture essential fatty acids, so you need to consume those good oils to ensure good health.

The best and simplest way to include good fats in the diet while avoiding bad ones is to use EFAs like flaxseed oil in salad dressing—also delicious on raw vegetables, on cooked grains and on whole grain bread. Flaxseed oil becomes unhealthy when heated, so cook with cold-pressed, extra-virgin olive oil, a healthy fat that can be heated without becoming unhealthy.

Nuts and seeds have a reputation for being high in fat. But they contain essential fatty acids that can help you with PMS and many illnesses. And, contrary to what many people believe, when nuts are consumed in moderation, studies have revealed that they actually lower body fat!

If you decrease the amount of saturated fat in your diet, you'll also dramatically reduce estrogen.[3] As you now know, high estrogen levels are a leading cause of PMS. The best—and also the easiest—way to cut down on the bad fats is to cut back on, or eliminate, animal products.

In addition to saturated fats, it is equally important to avoid trans-fatty acids, hydrogenated and partially hydrogenated oils which are found in many margarines, processed foods, packaged foods, baked goods and prepared salad dressings. To make a hydrogenated oil, a hydrogen molecule is added to the unsaturated oil, making it like a saturated fat. This change interferes with the body's ability to use the crucial essential fatty acids and actually makes the oil harmful to your health. Of all the oils to avoid, these are top of the list.

The diet recommendations discussed above will go a long way toward increasing your intake of good fats and decreasing the bad. When plant foods do contain fats, they are almost always healthy fats that will improve your body's function, including your immune system and brain function. They also provide countless other wonderful health benefits.

Reduce Simple Sugars and Refined Carbohydrates

Simple sugars are simply bad for PMS and to feel better we need to get them out of the diet as much as possible. Sugar impairs your body's ability to metabolize estrogen, so when you eat sugar, your estrogen levels go up. The more sugar you eat, the more severe your PMS symptoms will be.[4] PMS symptoms are more frequent in women on a high-sugar diet, and one study showed that eating a high-sugar diet was the most important factor in your chances of suffering from PMS.[5] Refined carbohydrates, like white flour, should also be reduced, since they are carbohydrates that have had all of the nutritional value of the grain removed, essentially leaving a simple sugar behind.

Sugar is not easy to cut out, though, right? Easier than you may think! You can eat all the fruit that you want instead, and soon you'll feel so great, and so free of cravings, it will easily be worth it. White sugar, brown sugar, molasses, honey, fructose on its own and simple carbohydrates (refined bread products and refined grains like white rice) should all be reduced since they contribute to PMS. A great alternative to processed sugars is stevia, a herbal sugar substitute that is even safe for diabetics. It is actually good for you! Flavor muffins, cookies, cakes and pies with fruit and stevia instead of sugar, and discover the many restaurants and cafes that now offer similar, healthy alternatives. Watch for labels that have hidden sources of sugar. They contain words like: sucrose, glucose, lactose, corn syrup, dextrose and maltose. Pretty much any word that ends in "ose" is a sugar.

Did you know that alcohol is a simple sugar? Try to cut back on it, or better yet, eliminate it. Alcohol increases estrogen levels, impairs liver function and makes PMS worse.

Equally dangerous is the classic premenstrual chocolate craving. Why do we crave chocolate? Probably because chocolate contains magnesium, and women with PMS often have low levels of magnesium. Yet chocolate is the food most likely to cause PMS symptoms.[6] It contains both sugar and caffeine, two things that are especially bad for women who suffer from PMS. Study after study continues to report these findings, despite all the recent hype about chocolate being good for you because it's rich in antioxidants. Try delicious unsweetened carob products instead.

Focus on what you can enjoy while you're balancing your hormones and leaving your PMS symptoms behind. Naturally occurring sugars, like the kinds found in fruits and vegetables, are good for you when they are consumed in their whole food form, that is, as a fruit or vegetable. When it comes to choosing carbs, whole grains just taste better and they are much healthier. Replace your white bread with brown, your white rice with brown and your white pasta with whole grain pasta. And still enjoy the foods you love. Look for restaurants that do the same.

Cut the Caffeine

If you suffer from breast tenderness, mood disorders, irritability, insomnia and depression during the days on which you have PMS, caffeine must be strictly avoided. Even one cup of coffee a day significantly aggravates PMS symptoms. Specifically, caffeine aggravates the psychological symptoms of PMS, like anxiety, depression and irritability. It also contributes to breast pain and tenderness. Even decaffeinated coffee, which still contains a small amount of caffeine, can bother women who are sensitive to caffeine. When caffeine is combined with sugar by women with PMS, disaster strikes. Watch for sources of hidden caffeine too, in pop, tea and chocolate. Instead, try a naturally decaffeinated green tea or other herbal teas like roasted dandelion or chicory root (coffee substitutes) to help you make the transition.

Improving Your Salt Ratio

Try to reduce your intake of salt. To make this easier, try shakers that contain salt alternatives; you can find these in health food stores. These substitutes are usually made of dried herbs and veggies and they taste great.

Salt can cause water retention, one of the leading problems women with PMS experience. Most North American diets are too high in sodium (salt) and too low in potassium. The recommended ratio of potassium to sodium is five to one, yet most people ingest twice as much salt as potassium. Fruits and vegetables are full of potassium, so the easiest way to correct this imbalance is to eat more of them. Particularly good sources of potassium are avocados, potatoes, tomatoes, lima beans, peaches, celery, bananas, carrots and spinach.

Eat More Soy

Soy foods contain phytoestrogens, which bind to estrogen receptor sites in your body and balance your estrogen levels. Phytoestrogens are only 2 percent as strong as your body's estrogen. If your estrogen is too low, as in menopause, phytoestrogens supply estrogen to receptor sites, thus increasing estrogen in your body. If your estrogen levels are too high, as in PMS, phytoestrogens prevent your body's estrogen from binding to receptors sites, thus lowering your body's estrogen.

Studies have shown that phytoestrogens prevent cancers, especially breast cancer. They're also good for fibroids, cysts, endometriosis and fibrocystic breast disease—all connected to high estrogen levels.

Soy comes in many forms: tempeh, tofu, soymilk, powder, pills and miso, to name but a few. There are also many convenient packaged foods, like soyburgers, soy hot dogs, luncheon slices, bacon and chili. Don't like soy, but want the health benefits of this amazing food? You can hide the taste of tofu in lots of dishes. Try pudding, cheesecake and spaghetti sauce made with soy.

Put the Green Back in Your Neighborhood

Grow green, buy green and eat green. Why?

Estrogen-mimicking chemicals called halogenated hydrocarbons have led to an increase in estrogen-related conditions such as PMS, fibroids and breast cancer.[7] These chemicals include toxic pesticides that, if ingested, stay in your body's fat cells.

So what can you do to avoid exposure to these harmful chemicals?

- Eat fewer dairy products and less meat because they contain high levels of pesticide residue.
- Don't spray pesticides/herbicides on your lawn, and encourage your neighbors to stop spraying. Sound impossible? I tried it. I distributed a flyer anonymously

in our neighborhood, describing the dangers of pesticides. Within a few weeks, several lawns displayed signs that said "chemical-free lawn." Some cities have seen the dangers and have enacted a ban on pesticides. Some of our neighbors actually share produce and talk about tips on how to grow things without pesticide.

- Buy organic produce or, better still, grow your own. Start small: a pot of basil. You'll see how fast it will catch on. You might soon have a whole garden growing.
- Use natural products—without chemicals—to clean your house, your clothes, your dishes, your car—and you. Check out health food stores: they have many great products.
- Wash your produce with a natural product that removes pesticides.
- Avoid storing foods in plastic containers; do not drink from plastic containers. Use glass instead. Plastics may cause increased estrogen levels.

Even if you cannot get organic produce where you live, it is still better to eat fruits and vegetables than to eat animal products. And the reason is simple: when you eat an apple, you are ingesting the pesticide of one apple; when you eat an animal product, you are ingesting all of the pesticides from all of the food eaten by that animal, and so the pesticide is in higher concentrations. And the standard diet of animals raised for food is loaded with pesticides and hormones. Also, plant foods are loaded with antioxidants that help the body to deal with the pesticide.

Eat Foods Rich in Sulfur

Sulfur is one of the key nutrients for eliminating excess estrogen from the body. So foods rich in sulfur help prevent PMS. Such foods include garlic, onions and beans. Or you can use methylsulfonylmethane (MSM), a sulfur-rich supplement.

Enjoy the Sunlight

Many women with PMS don't get enough natural sunlight. In one study, women were treated with two hours of bright light in the mornings: their symptoms were reversed.[8] Sunlight also helps prevent cancers, for example, breast and colon cancer. Get out in the sun and go for a walk in the early or later hours. It will be doubly good, as exercise helps PMS.

The Perfect PMS Diet

The perfect PMS diet is low in refined carbohydrates, salt, caffeine, alcohol, simple sugars, hydrogenated fats, trans fats and animal products. Chemicals should be shunned, as well as plastics.

It's full of wonderful flavors and includes lots of fiber and healthy fats from organic fruits, vegetables, whole grains, raw seeds, nuts and legumes. It focuses on soy and includes sulfur-rich foods like onions, garlic and beans. Essential fatty acids feature largely in the diet, and women should be out in the sunlight and exercising!

6

The Natural Approach to PMS: Herbs and Supplements

L et's start with some quick information about supplements, so you'll know what to use, when to use it and what to look for. There are many natural supplements available, and they can often be used together, so feel free to follow the sample protocol at the end of this chapter on your own. However, if you are taking medications, or have a serious underlying health condition, seek the help of a trained natural health-care practitioner.

How to Take Herbs and Supplements

Most often herbs are taken on an empty stomach and vitamins and minerals are taken with food. An empty stomach means half an hour before meals or two to three hours after meals.

Herbs come in pills, tinctures, extracts and loose as teas. In general, liquids are better absorbed. Some herbs are standardized, which means they contain a certain level of an active ingredient that is believed, or proven, to work best. Scientists like standardization because it ensures that the concentrations of certain ingredients are always the same, also that they are the same as those used in studies. Standardizing may cause certain ingredients in the herbs to be higher than in the herbs' natural state. Traditional herbalists often use nonstandardized herbs, as they prefer to use herbs in their unaltered natural state, where all the components are balanced in their natural proportions. Some products contain both in the same bottle, and I like these products and get good results using them clinically. Although I sometimes prefer one form over another, in general, I like both forms of herbs, and both are powerful and effective. To get good-quality herbs, buy a trusted brand, for example, one a practitioner has recommended. You can find herbs and supplements in health food stores, drugstores and supermarkets. Feel free to ask for help when you're shopping: sometimes the choices can be overwhelming. Loose dried herbs lose their potency within one to two years, though for some herbs, that time frame is less.

Infusions: An infusion is made by using the soft parts of the plant, like the flowers or leaves, brewed into a tea. You pour boiling water over the herb, cover it and let it stand for ten to twenty minutes. Strain and drink. The general rule of thumb is one teaspoon (5 mL) of dried herb for each cup (250 mL) of boiling water.

Decoctions: A decoction is made from the hard parts of the plant—the roots, bark and berries. To decoct an herb, put the dried herb in a stainless-steel or glass pot, pour cold water over it, cover, bring to a boil, then simmer. Some herbs need twenty minutes, some need an hour. Strain and drink. The rule of thumb is one teaspoon (5 mL) of dried herb for each cup (250 mL) of water.

Pills: Pills often contain just the powdered herb or a concentrated version of the herb called a solid extract.

Tinctures and Extracts: Liquids can be tinctures or extracts. Tinctures usually contain one part herb to five parts of a liquid solvent, usually alcohol or glycerin (1:5 concentration). A fluid extract is a stronger concentration: it is usually one part of the herb to one part liquid solvent (1:1 concentration). Extremely concentrated extracts can be as high as 50:1.

Many herbs can be used in all the different forms given. The choices are given here so that you will understand the dosages outlined in the coming chapters and have a choice as to which you prefer. Some prefer pills, some tinctures and some teas.

Queen of All Herbs for Women: Chastetree Berry (Vitex)

Chastetree berry is the most important herb for normalizing and regulating the menstrual cycle. The use of chastetree berry is not new: in Europe it is the best known herb for hormonal imbalances in women, and in Germany it has been studied repeatedly. It was used by the ancient Greeks for all kinds of menstrual problems, including heavy periods, lack of periods, lack of ovulation, frequent and infrequent periods and irregular periods. Today, it is used for all of the same reasons and is also much employed in treating PMS, menopause and painful periods. Pretty impressive for one little herb!

In Europe, chastetree berry is the number one herb to help relieve depression, cramps, mood swings, water retention, weight gain, and other PMS symptoms associated with an imbalance of the female hormones. Chastetree berry was rated in two German studies, including over 1,500 women, to be good or very good in the treatment of PMS. Over 90 percent of the women reported a complete cure or an improvement from their PMS symptoms.[1,2]

Recently, chastetree berry was tested in its first placebo-controlled study. One hundred and seventy women with PMS were given 20 mg of chastetree berry extract or a placebo for three menstrual cycles. There was a significantly greater reduction in symptom scores in the herb group, including symptoms of breast tenderness, bloating, headache, mood swing and irritability. Symptoms were reduced for 52 percent of the women by 50 percent or more, compared with only 24 percent of the placebo group.[3]

How exactly does chastetree berry work? Chastetree berry acts on a tiny area of the brain, called the hypothalamus, and on the pituitary glands. Chastetree berry increases the production of luteinizing hormone (LH) and slightly inhibits the release of follicle-stimulating hormone (FSH), thereby shifting the ratio of estrogen to progesterone. Herbalist David Hoffmann says chastetree berry has a normalizing effect on estrogen as "it will always enable what is appropriate to occur,"[4] although it does favor progesterone. A great deal of scientific research has confirmed that chastetree berry enhances the progesterone cycle in women. Chastetree berry also inhibits the pituitary gland's release of prolactin, particularly in times of stress, so the herb is particularly useful for prolactin excess (see page 17).

According to herbalist Michael Tierra, chastetree berry is the single most important herb for balancing emotion and mood before and during menstruation. As a herbalist, I have seen scores of women whose main symptoms of PMS were emotional instability use a combination of chastetree berry, liver herbs, vitamins and minerals and regain their emotional health after three months of following such programs.

Why three months? Chastetree berry is not a herb that works quickly. It takes time to normalize the cycle. Clinical evidence suggests that chastetree berry starts working after only ten days, but most herbalists suggest using chastetree berry for a minimum of three months, and preferably longer. Herbalist Christopher Hobbs says that long-lasting or permanent relief from PMS is actually possible after one year of chastetree berry therapy; he says if the imbalance has existed for a very long time, it may take up to two years to correct the underlying problem. Chastetree berry has been shown in research to not only balance the female hormones, but to actually cure PMS caused by abnormal levels of estrogen.

Wow, a possible cure, after years of women suffering.

Women with acne problems related to their periods should take note of this amazing herb. I have seen women who normally had very bad outbreaks prior to their periods achieve clearer skin after only three months of using chastetree berry and following a healthy, cleansing diet.

Dosage: 3 to 6 grams of the dried and ground berries three times a day. If you are using the tincture, take 30 drops three times a day. Chastetree berry is often standardized for 0.5 percent agnuside. If you are using a standardized tablet (this form is preferable), take 175 to 225 mg daily; if you are taking a standardized liquid extract, take ½ tsp (2 mL) a day.

Note

Some people say women on the pill should be careful when using chastetree berry if they do not wish to conceive, since it may interfere with the pill, although, to my knowledge, this problem has not occurred. The interaction is only speculative, and at least three recent studies found no negative interaction between the herb and the birth control pill.[5]

Licorice Root

Licorice root has been used for literally thousands of years for a variety of complaints, including PMS. Licorice works by lowering estrogen levels and raising progesterone levels. How does it do this? Our bodies contain an enzyme that breaks down progesterone; licorice prevents the enzyme from working. Like soy, licorice also has phytoestrogenic activity and can raise or lower the body's estrogen levels as needed, reducing PMS symptoms.

But that is not the only way that licorice can help women who suffer from PMS. It is also extremely helpful for water retention, which is sometimes caused by too much of the hormone aldosterone. Licorice binds to aldosterone receptors and blocks the hormone's effects. Since its activity is only one quarter as strong as the body's own aldosterone, the effect is to lower the overall levels in the body. This use of licorice may seem ironic, since it is better known for raising blood pressure by increasing sodium and water retention. The difference is in the part of the licorice you use: whole licorice root does not raise blood pressure, but isolated extracts of licorice do.[6]

To prevent problems with licorice, use only whole licorice root, and eat a diet high in potassium. (See the vegetarian diet discussed in Chapter 5.) Potassium lowers sodium and can lower blood pressure.

Licorice contains substances similar to adrenal cortical hormones, and so it can also be used to treat weak adrenal glands. One of the main functions of the adrenal glands is to deal with stress. So licorice is particularly useful for women who suffer from stress-related PMS symptoms.

Dosage: Licorice is best taken starting on day fourteen of the cycle and continuing until menstruation begins. If using the powder, take 1 to 2 grams three times a day; if using the fluid extract (1:1), take ½–1 tsp (2–4 mL) three times a day; if using the solid dry powdered extract (4:1), take 250 to 500 mg three times a day.

Black Cohosh

Black cohosh was once believed to be phytoestrogenic, but now it seems it is not.[7] Instead, its nervine-relaxing properties make it useful for women who suffer from stress induced by PMS. In one study of 135 women, a black coshosh extract was found to significantly reduce feelings of depression, anxiety, tension and mood swings.[8]

Black cohosh has been used for centuries by North America's First Nations people; later it was used by early colonists to treat a wide variety of women's health complaints. The word "cohosh" comes from the First Nations Algonquian people, and it means "rough root."

This herb has been standardized to contain 1 mg of triterpenes calculated as 27-deoxyacteine per tablet, and it is the number-one natural seller for treating menopause. The standardized extract of black cohosh has also shown significant benefits in treating PMS.

Dosage: To treat PMS, take one tablet of the extract once or twice daily. This will give you 2 to 4 mg of 27-deoxyacteine. If you use the nonstandardized version, take 3 to 9 grams a day, or 10 to 30 drops of the tincture three times a day.

Dong Quai

Dong quai is used for almost every female health-related complaint and is used specifically for treating the uterus. It is of special use to those suffering from cramping or weakness during menstruation, lack of periods, abnormal periods and anemia from heavy flow. Dong quai is also good for women with PMS who also experience cramping.

In Asia, dong quai is held in very high regard, second only to ginseng. It is mainly used by women. Just how does dong quai work? Research suggests that it tones the uterus by increasing uterine contractions, then encouraging uterine relaxation. Studies have also shown that dong quai increases the weight of the uterus, increases the blood flow to it, and reduces blockages that cause sluggish menstrual flow (a sluggish flow can create PMS symptoms and pain). Dong quai also causes the liver and the uterus to use more glucose.

Dong quai is usually given fourteen days after menstruation has begun and is taken until bleeding begins. Keep taking it throughout the period if you feel pain. It should not be used by women who experience heavy bleeding during their periods, although they can take it up until the time that their periods begin.

Dosage: 4 to 7 grams a day. As a tea, take 1 cup (250 mL) three times a day; as a tincture, take ½ to 1 tsp (2 mL–4 mL) three times a day; of the fluid extract, take ¼ tsp (1 mL) three times a day.

Progesterone Cream

This is one of the supplements most recommended by naturally oriented doctors. PMS is believed to be caused by an estrogen dominance, and many naturally oriented practitioners have successfully used progesterone creams to treat PMS. John R. Lee, MD, in his book *What Your Doctor May Not Tell You about Menopause*, reports success using a progesterone cream with many of his patients who have PMS. Specifically, he writes that patients report an improvement in their symptoms, including water retention and weight gain.

Dosage: The dosage for progesterone cream is specific to each individual, so visit a health-care practitioner.

Dandelion Root and Other Liver Detoxifiers

Liver herbs are important in treating PMS since they help clear out a clogged liver—think of it as a clogged drain—allowing it to unload its toxic load. Liver support is also important for women with PMS since it helps to rid the body of candida (an overgrowth of bad intestinal flora), another possible cause of PMS. The liver is also responsible for breaking estrogen down into a safer form.

There are many liver herbs that can be used: dandelion root, milk thistle, yellow dock, Oregon grape root, black radish, artichoke, boldo and many others. These herbs encourage the production and excretion of bile. They detoxify a wide range of substances from the body, including chemicals, excess estrogen, and pesticides. Milk thistle and artichoke even rebuild damaged liver cells. Many health food stores carry a variety of liver-cleansing herbs.

Dosage: This will depend on which herbs you use, but in general, use 30 to 40 drops of good-quality liver tinctures, for example, dandelion root, milk thistle, yellow dock and Oregon grape root. Take the drops three to four times a day on an empty stomach. Or you can drink three cups of liver herbs tea a day.

B6

Vitamin B6 has become a popular choice for women with PMS. Even many conventional doctors and health centers now know about its effectiveness and recommend it along with chastetree berry. This change is good news: more women are finding real help for PMS, and PMS is starting to be seen as a real illness.

Originally, B6 was used to treat depression caused by the birth control pill. The treatment was so successful researchers began to investigate B6's use for treating PMS. Since 1975, there have been at least a dozen double-blind clinical trials. A 1999 analysis of the best quality studies of B6 concluded that the vitamin is more than twice as likely as a placebo to help women who suffer from PMS.[9] For example, in one double-blind study, 84 percent of women who used B6 experienced improved symptoms.[10]

Some women are unable to convert B6 into its active form, so the vitamin doesn't help them as much. These women may lack vitamin B2 and magnesium: nutrients necessary to convert B6. Some women may need to add a wider-spectrum nutritional supplement to receive the benefits of B6.

B6 is a diuretic, so it can help relieve the water retention many women with PMS experience. B6 has also been reported to alleviate symptoms such as nervousness, irritability, depression, bloating, breast tenderness, weight gain, and skin and digestive problems. B6 is believed to increase the synthesis of several neurotransmitters in the brain, including serotonin.

B6 also helps PMS in other ways, since B6 and magnesium interact with each other. B6 seems to increase the accumulation of magnesium in body cells, and without B6, magnesium cannot get into the cells. Several studies show that B6 and magnesium taken together in a multivitamin-mineral supplement can dramatically reduce PMS symptoms.

> **Dosage**: A safe dosage of B6 for treating PMS is 50 to 200 mg daily, taken with food. Studies indicate that the liver can't handle more than 50 mg of B6 at a time, so if you are using the larger amount, take it in divided doses. Take a B-complex as well, to avoid causing any imbalances. B-vitamins also help with mood and are involved in many different bodily functions.

Magnificent Magnesium

The typical western diet is chronically low in magnesium. And, interestingly, a low level of magnesium is an important causative factor in PMS. Several studies have shown that magnesium levels are consistently lower in women with PMS than in women without.[11]

A magnesium deficiency may account for a wide range of PMS symptoms, such as headaches, fatigue, irritability, heart palpitations, stress, mood swings, nervous sensitivity, aches and pains and a lower pain threshold. Clinical trials with magnesium show a reduction in PMS symptoms. One trial showed that magnesium reduced nervousness in 89 percent of the women, breast tenderness in 96 percent and weight gain in 95 percent.[12] Other studies have shown an extremely significant reduction in mood changes.

 Dosage: Take 12 mg of magnesium for every 2.2 pounds (1 kg) of body weight to treat PMS. The best forms to take are aspartate, citrate, malate, succinate and fumarate: all are well absorbed, utilized and tolerated. Take every day, with food.

Getting Your Calcium

Like so many others, have you been brainwashed into thinking that calcium is only found in dairy products? This is not at all true. So where can you get calcium? Simple. Whole grains, deep leafy greens, sea vegetables, nuts and seeds, herbs and legumes are all good sources of calcium, and they are all components of a healthy vegetarian diet. Try to eat at least one serving of dark green leafy vegetables a day: kale, chard, beet greens, spinach, mustard greens and watercress are good choices. Another good source of calcium is sesame seeds; you might try tahini, a spread made from brown sesame seeds that's loaded with calcium.

Dairy products are high in calcium—but they're also high in animal protein and phosphorus, two substances that can leach calcium from the body. In fact, high milk consumption is linked to PMS. Both dairy products and animal protein should be reduced or eliminated in women with premenstrual syndrome.[11]

Unlike calcium from dairy products, taking a calcium supplement helps PMS. Double-blind studies have found that 1,200 mg of calcium daily can reduce the symptoms of PMS by 48 percent.[13] Other studies show that women with PMS improve with calcium and manganese supplements. These women reported improvement in mood, concentration and behavior. And, most recently, it has now been shown that calcium can not only help you once you have PMS, but can actually help you to avoid it. Women with the highest intake of calcium are 30 percent less likely to suffer from PMS.[14]

 Dosage: For women with PMS, 1,000 to 1,500 mg of calcium balanced with magnesium (see above) with food every day.

Vitamin E

Supplementing with vitamin E helps reduce breast tenderness, nervous tension, headaches, fatigue, depression, anxiety, food cravings, weight gain and insomnia.

And the results are quick. One study showed that women experienced relief from PMS symptoms after about three months of vitamin E therapy.[15]

🌿 **Dosage**: Take 400 IU per day with food. Only use natural vitamin E. Look at the fine print on the bottle. If the vitamin E is natural, the name on the bottle will start with "d-," as in d-alpha-tocopherol. If it's synthetic, it will start with "dl-." Good forms of natural vitamin E include d-alpha-tocopherol; even better are, d-alpha-tocopheryl acetate and d-alpha-tocopheryl succinate. There is more than one member of the vitamin E family, and getting your alpha-tocopherol mixed with beta, delta and gamma tocopherols may even be better.

Zinc

Studies consistently show that women with PMS have lower levels of zinc than healthy women. When zinc is low, levels of prolactin go up, and when levels of prolactin go up, PMS is worse. Women with elevated prolactin levels absolutely must take zinc to treat PMS.

Zinc can be particularly helpful for women who suffer from bad acne during their periods: zinc encourages healing, strengthens the immune system and prevents scarring. I find that women who suffer from acne can often reduce or eliminate the acne altogether by taking zinc and chastetree berry while they also clean out and rebalance their digestive systems. Even women who have tried all of the conventional remedies (antibiotics and topical creams) to no avail tend to respond to this program.

🌿 **Dosage:** 25 to 50 mg of zinc citrate a day. Zinc should be balanced with copper at a ratio of ten to one, so you can take 2 to 3 mg of copper daily, unless a hair mineral analysis indicates a chronically low zinc to copper ratio. When you take large doses of zinc, you may also want to take folic acid.[16]

Essential Fatty Acids

Ninety percent of all Americans are deficient in essential fatty acids. That is a staggering number, and it means we don't get enough EFAs from our diets. Yet EFAs are important—life without them is impossible, because they're involved in numerous bodily functions. More than sixty different illnesses are treated with EFAs, and that is a conservative number. So it is not surprising that PMS would also benefit from EFA supplementation.

Women with PMS have deficiencies or abnormalities of essential fatty acids.[17] One example is gamma-linolenic acid (GLA), the EFA most women with PMS are deficient in. To make GLA, your body requires zinc, B6 and magnesium, nutrients that are already low if you have PMS.

There is more than one kind of EFA. While the research on treating PMS with sources of GLA, like evening primrose oil (omega 6), is largely negative, the research on treating women with PMS with omega 3 oils, like flaxseed, is better. For this reason, it is a good idea for those who suffer from PMS to supplement their diet with flaxseed oil, or a mixture of omega 3 and 6 rather than just GLA.

Dosage: 1 tablespoon (15 mL) or more a day of flaxseed oil (primarily a source of omega 3) or try a two-to-one ratio of omega 3 to 6, with a source of GLA (like evening primrose oil) as part of the mixture.

5-HTP

According to Anita Rapkin, MD, women with PMS typically experience a reduction in serotonin levels during the last half of the menstrual cycle. Serotonin helps to induce sleep, prevents migraines, anxiety and depression and helps to stabilize both weight and mood: all symptoms of PMS.

Conventional doctors often prescribe Prozac to women with PMS who are depressed or moody, since Prozac elevates serotonin levels. Yet Prozac has caused many deaths due to suicide; as well, prescription drugs are expensive and have numerous unpleasant side effects, like dry mouth, fatigue, anxiety and loss of libido.

5-HTP (a naturally occurring substance) increases serotonin naturally and safely and can be of huge benefit to women whose PMS symptoms are caused by low serotonin levels. 5-HTP also raises levels of endorphins, your body's natural painkillers.[18] Low levels of endorphins in women with PMS contribute to mood problems and pain.

Dosage: 50 to 100 mg three times a day as long as needed. 5-HTP is a safe alternative to drugs and is without side effects, but it's not easy to monitor and diagnose depression in yourself. So take 5-HTP under the supervision of a natural health-care practitioner. 5-HTP should not be taken with selective serotonin reuptake inhibitors (SSRI antidepressants), or other serotonin-producing substances, without supervision.

St. John's Wort

Women with PMS who suffer from depression may want to try St. John's wort, the best antidepressant herb. St. John's wort has consistently proven itself to be better than Prozac and other SSRI antidepressants in controlled studies. In a recent study, people with major depression were given St. John's wort, Prozac or a placebo. Depression scores improved significantly more in the St. John's wort group than in the Prozac group, according to the Hamilton Depression Scale.[19] St. John's wort can also help increase deep sleep.

🌿 **Dosage:** 300 mg of standardized St. John's wort extract three times a day. Don't use with SSRI antidepressants, or other serotonin-producing substances, without supervision.

Kava and Passionflower

Women who suffer anxiety during PMS may want to try kava, one of the very best herbs for anxiety. If kava is unavailable, try passionflower, which is also excellent for anxiety. An exciting double-blind study compared passionflower to the benzodiazepine drug Oxazepam. (Benzodiazepines are the most commonly used drugs for anxiety.) The passionflower worked just as well, but was actually even better than the drug because it caused fewer side effects.[20] Both passionflower and kava help with sleep.

🌿 **Dosage:** 45 to 70 mg of kavalactones three times a day on an empty stomach. Or 40 drops of passionflower three or four times per day, or as needed, on an empty stomach.

Valerian Root and Other Sleep Aids

If you're having difficulty sleeping, try valerian root, which works better than benzodiazepines for insomnia.[21] Benzodiazepines are the most commonly used medications for insomnia. In studies of insominia, valerian eased anxiety as well as benzodiazepines.

Other good choices include hops, skullcap, lemon balm, lemon verbena and wild oats. These herbs will help you fall asleep faster and encourage a deep and natural sleep without a morning hangover. They can also be used for anxiety.

🌿 **Dosage:** 150 to 300 mg (standardized for 0.8 percent valeric acid) thirty minutes before retiring. For anxiety and sleep issues, try hops, skullcap, lemon balm, lemon verbena or wild oats in dropper form: 40 drops, three to four times per day.

SAMe

If you suffer from depression, anxiety or pain, try SAMe. It is one of the best new nutrients for increasing serotonin and melatonin, helping you to feel less depressed, less anxious and allowing you to sleep better. It also relieves certain kinds of pain by increasing serotonin. As a bonus, it detoxifies the liver too.

🌿 **Dosage:** 400 to 1,500 mg, in divided dosages, started slowly and increasing every two weeks as needed. Don't use with SSRI antidepressants, or other serotonin-producing substances, without supervision.

Acidophilus and Bifidus

Try using probiotics—acidophilus and bifidus—to reduce excess estrogen. When you reduce excess estrogen, you reduce PMS symptoms. Probiotics also encourage the liver to detoxify, and they're a great help for women who have acne.

Dosage: 2 to 20 billion live cells every day on an empty stomach. The higher dosage is usually only used for short periods of time.

Wide-Spectrum Multivitamin and Mineral

Women with PMS should take a wide-spectrum multivitamin and mineral. A double-blind crossover study done in 1985 looked at women who used a multivitamin that met or exceeded the recommended daily allowance (RDA) for most nutrients. Women on a multivitamin reported feeling better on the supplement during their cycles.[22] A multivitamin can also help correct underlying nutritional deficiencies.

Finally an End to PMS

PMS can be helped with a natural, comprehensive program that accounts for all the factors involved. Working with a natural health practitioner is often a good way to be sure you're taking a multifaceted approach. The suggestions given in this book are designed to help women help themselves and encourage women to take charge of their health. The suggestions are safe and effective ways to help women get over PMS. Now let's break it down and make it easy to get started.

The PMS Protocol

Start with the dietary suggestions in Chapter 5.

Chastetree Berry: *Take 3 to 6 grams of the dried and ground berries three times a day. If you are using the tincture, take 30 drops three times a day on an empty stomach, before breakfast, lunch and dinner. Chastetree berry is often standardized for 0.5 percent agnuside. If you are using a standardized tablet (this form is preferable), take 175 to 225 mg daily; if you are taking a standardized liquid extract, take ½ tsp (2mL) a day. For many women, this alone may be enough to correct PMS.*

Multivitamin and mineral: *All women should take a multivitamin and mineral. Take one a day with food.*

Flaxseed oil: *Add 1 tablespoon (15 mL) to your salad dressing.*

Calcium, magnesium: *These are important, especially if you have emotional symptoms and cramping. Take 1,200 mg of calcium and 600 to 800 mg of magnesium*

continued

every day with food. Check the dosage of your multivitamin/mineral, some calcium and magnesium are already in it. All women should take these two nutrients for their bones.

This may be all you need to bring your body back into balance. However, you may also want to consider some additional support:

Liver and digestive support: *Take probiotics—between 2 and 20 billion active cultures—per day on an empty stomach. The easiest way is to take the probiotics as soon as you wake up or right before you go to bed. Take probiotics for at least three to six months. This will clean your liver and lower the bad forms of estrogen.*

Liver tonic: *Clean your liver with one of the liver herbs: yellow dock, boldo, artichoke, dandelion root, Oregon grape root or milk thistle. Take 40 drops of any one, or more, of these three times per day on an empty stomach.*

Additional Help

Water Retention

If water retention and breast tenderness are still issues after three months, take 50 mg of vitamin B6 three times a day with food.

You could also add in licorice: It's best to start on day fourteen of your cycle and continue until menstruation begins. If you use the powder, take 1 to 2 grams three times a day; if you use the fluid extract (1:1), take ½–1 tsp (2-4 mL) three times a day; if you use the solid dry powdered extract (4:1), take 250 to 500 mg three times a day. Always take licorice on an empty stomach.

Depression

For depression, use chastetree berry and/or black cohosh. Add either SAMe, 5-HTP or St. John's wort. Do not take SAMe, St. Johns' wort and 5-HTP together without professional supervision, as you might get too much serotonin.

- *Chastetree berry: The usual dosage of chastetree berry is 3 to 6 grams of the dried and ground berries three times a day; of the tincture, 30 drops three times a day. Chastetree berry is often standardized for 0.5 percent agnuside. If you are using a standardized tablet, take 175 to 225 mg daily; if a liquid extract, take ½ teaspoon (2 mL) a day.*
- *Black cohosh: take one tablet of the extract once or twice daily. This will give you 2 to 4 mg of 27-deoxyacteine. If you use the nonstandardized version, take 3 to 9 grams a day, or 10 to 30 drops of the tincture three times a day.*
- *SAMe: 400 to 1,500 mg, in divided dosages, started slowly and increasing every two weeks as needed. Don't use with SSRI antidepressants, or other serotonin-producing substances, without supervision.*

- 5-HTP: 50 to 100 mg three times a day as long as needed. Don't use with SSRI anti-depressants, or other serotonin-producing substances, without supervision.
- St. John's wort: 300 mg of standardized St. John's wort extract three times a day. Don't use with SSRIs, or other serotonin-producing substances, without supervision.

Anxiety

To treat anxiety, add kava, and/or 5-HTP, passionflower or valerian to your daily protocol.

- Kava: 45 to 70 mg of kavalactones three times a day.
- 5-HTP: 50 to 100 mg three times a day as long as needed. Don't use with SSRI anti-depressants, or other serotonin-producing substances, without supervision.
- Passionflower: 40 drops three or four times per day, or as needed, on an empty stomach.
- Valerian: 150 to 300 mg standardized for 0.8 percent valeric acid thirty minutes before retiring.

Insomnia

To improve sleep problems, add any of: 5-HTP, St. John's wort, valerian, lemon verbena, lemon balm, hops or skullcap. Some herbs in this category can be combined, but you are best to do that only with a practitioner, as both St. John's wort and 5-HTP increase serotonin and should be monitored.

- 5-HTP: 50 to 100 mg three times a day as long as needed. Don't use with SSRI anti-depressants, or other serotonin-producing substances, without supervision.
- St. John's wort: 300 mg of standardized St. John's wort extract three times a day. Don't use with SSRIs, or other serotonin-producing substances, except with supervision.
- Valerian: 150 to 300 mg standardized for 0.8 percent valeric acid thirty minutes before retiring.
- Lemon verbena: as an infused tea before bed.
- Lemon balm: in dropper form, 40 drops three to four times per day.
- Hops: in dropper form, 40 drops three to four times per day.
- Skullcap: in dropper form, 40 drops three to four times per day.

Acne

For acne use 25 to 50 mg of zinc balanced with 2 to 3 mg of copper, as needed, with food. The chastetree berry and probiotics you are already taking may also help.

Feel free to experiment with the different options available: try the possibilities suggested in this chapter to alleviate any symptoms you may have. If after some time you decide

continued

you still need some help, try seeking an herbalist or other natural health practitioner. Some women feel more comfortable working with someone right from the beginning.

Now you know how to safely and effectively treat your PMS and are probably excited about getting started. So go right ahead—that is what this book is designed to help you with. And with a little time and effort, change will come, and you will be feeling so great you'll wonder why you didn't do it before.

7

Dysmenorrhea (Painful Periods)

I t's that time of the month again, and already you're starting to dread the pain your period will bring, the terrible cramping. But there is a way to avoid the pain. With a little work, you'll hardly even know your period has started: the cramping will be gone.

I do not say this lightly. I used to suffer terribly from cramping during the first two days of my period: so much so that despite the side effects of Naproxen, I took it anyway. I didn't know what else to do. Help for me came from herbs, supplements and acupuncture, and now my periods are virtually pain-free.

Hypochondriacs?

At one time, women who suffered from painful periods were thought to be hypochondriacs or unable to tolerate normal pain. In the 1950s, the literature was filled with the message that period pain was psychological, that it was caused by unhappiness about being a women. Now, fortunately, it is recognized as a medical condition that can be debilitating and that can prevent women from leading a normal life.

How Prevalent Is Dysmenorrhea?

As many as 60 percent of all women suffer from painful periods. For as many as 10 percent, the pain is so severe it's incapacitating. Approximately sixty million work hours are lost each year in the United States alone because of painful periods!

Symptoms

Period pain is caused by cramping in the abdomen, specifically the uterus, and often affects the lower back. Sometimes it disturbs the bowel. Women can also experience a reduced tolerance for pain.

Other common symptoms include vomiting, fatigue, bowel changes, nausea, headaches, dizziness and fainting. These symptoms occur partly because the uterus is so full and congested, since the blood has not yet begun to flow, that the bowels can be affected. Stool and urine are often not fully emptying.

Hormonal changes are involved, as is the liver.

Dysmenorrhea can also cause bloating, breast tenderness, weight gain and irritability. Confusing, isn't it? Sounds a lot like PMS. The main difference is that the symptoms of dysmenorrhea typically don't start until your period starts, or just before it; PMS can start anywhere from day fourteen onward, and can have more symptoms.

With dysmenorrhea, pain is typically felt prior to, or on the first and second day of, the period. It is often relieved when the main part of the blood has flowed.

Causes

Structural causes must be ruled out first. There are many, such as endometriosis, fibroids, infection, structural abnormalities and cysts. The suggestions given here are still helpful even if the cause is structural, although, obviously, the structural problems would need to be addressed.

Abnormal Prostaglandin Production

If there is no obvious structural problem, then the pain could be a result of abnormal prostaglandin production, which can cause pain and inflammation. Cramps can be caused by high levels of the hormone prostaglandin F2 alpha in the menstrual blood. When this hormone is released into the blood stream, the uterus goes into spasm, causing cramping. Obese women, women who have longer cycles, women who began their cycles at a young age and women who smoke are at greater risk for this problem.

Other Causes

Contributing factors include: a sluggish liver, hormonal imbalance, stress, poor fitness, poor blood flow, low calcium, low magnesium and poor eating habits and low thyroid. Behavioral and psychological factors are also contributing factors. Treatment is aimed at correcting these underlying problems.

Dietary Factors

Reduce Inflammatory Foods

Your diet should focus on whole foods, vegetables, grains, legumes, nuts and seeds; try to limit hydrogenated and saturated fats. Be sure to increase fiber to keep stool soft and moving—constipation makes dysmenorrhea worse.

Animal fats and animal proteins cause an increase in the pain-producing prostaglandins; essential fatty acids from flaxseed oil reduce the inflammation and pain. So eat that delicious flaxseed oil!

Clean Up Your Diet

At your own pace, reduce or eliminate coffee, alcohol, chocolate, soft drinks, sugar and refined carbohydrates from your diet. All these items leach out the minerals and essential fatty acids that promote a strong reproductive system. Also reduce or eliminate salt and animal protein, which contribute to dysmenorrhea.

Eat from the Sea

A low thyroid can contribute to dysmenorrhea. Include sea vegetables in your diet: they provide minerals, especially iodine, which can help to regulate an underactive thyroid. Sea vegetables include kelp, hijiki, nori and dulse. Look for them in health food stores and Asian markets. Try a seaweed salad or vegetable sushi.

The Role of Stress

Stress causes cramping. Many natural health practitioners believe that women who lead unbalanced lives, which do not sufficiently address their needs for peace, fulfillment and joy, are prime candidates for cramping.

Conventional Treatments

Cramps are often treated with nonsteroidal anti-inflammatory drugs (NSAIDs), for example, Naproxen, and birth control pills. NSAIDs block inflammatory prostaglandins but can have numerous side effects. The birth control pill prevents ovulation, and therefore it can prevent the symptoms associated with hormonal changes. However, it is not always completely effective in blocking pain. (Side effects of both drugs are described in Chapter 5.)

But there is a better safe and effective way to get rid of cramping. And it can be quite simple.

Herbs that Help

There are a lot of fabulous ways to reduce period pain. All these treatments work effectively. To learn how to treat yourself safely, effectively and naturally—and without unwanted side effects—read on.

Cramp Bark and Black Haw

These two herbs are considered perhaps the best relief for painful periods. They work by relaxing the smooth muscle of the uterus. Cramp bark can decrease the spasming of the cervical neck; First Nations people use black haw for female cramping.

Dosage: 40 drops of one or each three times per day on an empty stomach. For intense cramping, take cramp bark every half hour until the pain subsides.

Dong Quai

This herb brings warmth into the pelvic region and encourages blood flow, so it's very helpful in relieving cramping caused by cold or by reduced blood flow. It should not be used once the bleeding begins if you have heavy bleeding. Dong quai is one of the best herbs for relieving the pain of cramps.

Dosage: 40 drops three times per day on an empty stomach. It is best used starting on day fourteen and right into your period, if your flow is not too heavy, until the pain subsides.

Ginger

Ginger brings warmth to the abdomen and can help to relieve the pain. It also is an antispasmodic that can help to relieve the spasming. For those who suffer from nausea during their periods, ginger can help to alleviate this problem as well. It alleviates intestinal gas and helps to correct bowel functions.

Dosage: Ginger can be taken as a tea, and is very nice this way. One 500 mg capsule dissolved in one cup of hot water two to three times per day on an empty stomach. You can also take ginger pills (500 mg), two to three times per day on an empty stomach.

Ginger Foment

Ginger can also be applied as a foment to the abdominal region to help ease pain and inflammation and to restore blood circulation to the area. To make a foment, grate 2 ounces of fresh ginger in 1 pint of boiled water. Let stand covered for ten to twenty minutes. The water should turn yellow. Dip a cloth into the mixture and apply hot to the abdomen or lower back. Cover with a towel and a hot water bottle. Leave on until it cools and repeat as needed. Be careful not to burn yourself

Black Cohosh, Blue Cohosh

Black cohosh and blue cohosh are commonly used to relieve menstrual pains. Black cohosh is a powerful antispasmodic; it relaxes the body and eases cramping. Blue cohosh brings blood into the abdomen, thus easing congestion and pain. The two are often combined with chamomile, raspberry leaves and ginger.

Dosage: 40 drops of one or each three times per day on an empty stomach.

Motherwort

Motherwort is a powerful antispasmodic and nervine that can be particularly beneficial to women who experience cramping. It is often combined with dong quai and cramp bark for this purpose.

Dosage: 40 drops three times per day on an empty stomach.

Pennyroyal

The oil of the pennyroyal plant is not taken internally; use it as a rub for your lower abdomen. It brings blood flow into the area.

Dosage: Rub 2 to 10 drops (or less) on the abdomen as needed. Use a carrier oil, for example, almond oil or olive oil, if desired.

Hormone Balance for Cramps: Chastetree Berry

Taken over time, chastetree berry will correct an underlying hormonal imbalance and help to reduce cramping. (See page 38 for dosage and frequency.)

Clean Your Liver

Herbs like blessed thistle, milk thistle, yellow dock and dandelion root are used to clear out a clogged and sluggish liver. The liver is almost always involved in menstrual irregularities (see Chapter 3). Traditional oriental medicine attributes many menstrual problems to blocked liver *qi* (energy), so it is a good idea to clean and unblock the liver. These herbs are wonderful for your liver; use whichever you can find, or try combining them.

Dosage: 40 drops of one or each herb three times per day on an empty stomach.

Herbs to Relax You and Your Uterus: Valerian, Hops, and Linden

Herbs like hops, skullcap, linden, valerian, chamomile and lemon balm help to relax tension and can ease cramping. Valerian is an antispasmodic; linden flower can relieve headaches—including migraine headaches—associated with menstrual problems. Try any one of these, or combine them.

Dosage: 40 drops of one or each three to four times per day on an empty stomach. I particularly like using valerian and chamomile together: 40 drops of valerian, four times per day, in a cup of strongly infused chamomile tea.

Bromelain

Bromelain, which comes from pineapple, is one of the best herbs for period cramping. It helps to relax the smooth muscles of the uterus and reduces cramping. It's also an anti-inflammatory.

Dosage: One 500 mg capsule three times per day on an empty stomach.

Other Useful Herbs

Other useful herbs include raspberry leaf, yarrow, squaw vine, rosemary, nettle and prickly ash. They are often combined with the previously mentioned herbs and are given here as further choices, if more help is needed. Also this way, if you choose a formula that has one or more of these herbs in it, you will know it is a good choice.

Essential Fatty Acids

You'll find a full discussion on dietary factors in Chapter 5. For painful periods, it is especially important that you take at least one tablespoon of flaxseed oil per day. Other helpful nutrients for converting these good oils into powerful antispasmodics and anti-inflammatories include B6, zinc, magnesium, vitamin C and niacin, a kind of B vitamin. You can get all of these in a good quality multivitamin and mineral formula.

Vitamins, Minerals and Other Useful Supplements

Calcium and Magnesium

Blood calcium levels begin to drop prior to menstruation. Low levels of blood calcium are characterized by muscle cramps, water retention and aches, among other problems. In other words, low calcium levels help to cause dysmenorrhea.

Magnesium is not only important as an aid to calcium absorption, it also helps to reduce sensitivity to pain. Low levels of both calcium and magnesium tend to be found in women with dysmenorrhea.[1]

Dosage: 1,200 to 1,500 mg of calcium with food (preferably dinner), along with 600 to 800 mg of magnesium. You can get them together in one formula.

B6, B3 (Niacin) and B-Complex

When taken together, B6 and a B-complex—all of the Bs in one formula—reduce the intensity and the duration of cramping.[2] Clinical studies show that niacin (vitamin B3) is more than 87 percent effective in relieving menstrual cramps.[3] It may be that it acts as a vasodilator of the uterus, reducing the pain. Vitamin C and flavonoids, such as rutin, have been shown to enhance the effectiveness of niacin(B3) in relieving pain by enhancing the vasodilating effect of the niacin (B3).[4]

Dosage: 50 mg of B-complex three times per day with food; 50 mg of B6 three times per day with food.

Vitamin E

Taking 200 to 800 IU of vitamin E can help relieve dysmenorrhea. Up to 70 percent of women experience relief using vitamin E.[5] In a double-blind study, teenage girls with dysmenorrhea were given either 500 IU of vitamin E or a placebo for five days, beginning two days before menstruation. The girls taking the vitamin E experienced significant relief from menstrual pain.[6] In a second study, girls were given only 400 IU of vitamin E; they still had less pain, the pain didn't last as long and they lost less blood.[7]

Dosage: 200 to 800 IU of natural-sourced vitamin E with food each day. Start with the lower dosage and work your way up in 100 IU increments every two weeks, as needed. If you take blood thinners, please work with a natural healer.

MSM (MethylSufonylMethane)

Although MSM is not typically mentioned as a treatment for dysmenorrhea, I have found, clinically and personally, that it offers a great deal of relief for cramping caused by inflammation. MSM, a sulfur compound, is an anti-inflammatory and a painkiller and is typically used for joint problems and for rebuilding the gut. It also helps stop muscle spasms.

Dosage: 1,000 to 1,500 mg once per day.

SAMe and 5-HTP

Both SAMe and 5-HTP can also help by increasing serotonin, making you less sensitive to pain.

Dosage: 50 to 100 mg of 5-HTP—without another serotonin drug or herb unless under supervision—three times per day, or 200 to 400 mg; of SAMe. Watch for serotonin reactions. SAMe can be slowly increased to much higher dosages: 1,200 to 1,500 mg; however, it is a good idea to work with a healer to establish the best dosage for you and to watch that your serotonin does not get too high.

Supportive Therapies

Some women find that heat helps as a treatment for dysmenorrhea; some prefer cold. Traditional Chinese medicine says our preference has much to do with our body type. Those who prefer heat have a cold body type, and those who prefer cold have a hot body type. Use heat or cold in their many forms where appropriate.

Another useful remedy is the sitz bath: you sit in alternating buckets of hot and cold water, finishing with cold. I know—it sounds horrendous. But it is remarkably effective, so don't be afraid to give it a try!

Or try a castor-oil pack. Heat the castor oil and make a foment, then apply it to your abdomen for one hour, as with the ginger pack.

Progesterone cream may also be helpful. If progesterone cream interests you, see a practitioner to get a dosage specific to your individual needs.

Further helpful treatments or factors include acupuncture, avoidance of food allergens, improving digestive function, avoiding tampons and IUDs, and getting more exercise.

Finally an End to Painful Periods

Given a little time and effort, painful periods can be stopped. You can start by using the Protocol for Painful Cramping as a guide.

The Protocol for Painful Cramping

Follow the dietary suggestions given in this chapter and in Chapter 5. Also work to reduce stress. Acupuncture is a great way to do this, and it also is great for cramping.

Cramp bark: *40 drops of the tincture or liquid extract three to four times per day on an empty stomach, or every half-hour until pain diminishes.*

Calcium and magnesium: *1,200 mg of calcium with food (preferably dinner) and 600 mg of magnesium with food every day. You can get them together in one formula.*

Flaxseed oil: *One tablespoon (15 mL) daily.*

This may be all you need to bring your body into balance. However, you may also want to consider some additional support:

Bromelain: *500 mg capsule three times per day on an empty stomach.*

Dong quai: *40 drops three times per day from day fourteen of your cycle on. Take on an empty stomach.*

continued

*A*dditional Help

Vitamin E: *200 to 800 IU per day with food.*

B-complex and B6: *50 mg of each three times per day with food.*

Motherwort: *40 drops three to four times per day on an empty stomach.*

Blue cohosh and black cohosh: *40 drops of one or each three times per day on an empty stomach.*

Valerian: *40 drops three times per day on an empty stomach.*

Liver herbs: *dandelion root, yellow dock, and boldo; 40 drops of one or each three times per day on an empty stomach.*

SAMe: *200 to 400 mg three times per day with no other serotonin-increasing drug or herb, unless directed by a practioner. Higher dosages are used (see above).*

5-HTP: *50 to 100 mg three times per day with no other serotonin-increasing drug or herb, unless directed by a practioner.*

Castor oil pack: *Try this several times throughout the month to keep your system clean and clear.*

*T*ip

Chamomile tea: *I love to drink chamomile tea. You can have four cups a day. Use 1 tsp (5 mL) dried chamomile per 1 cup (250 mL) of boiling water; cover and let stand for about 20 minutes, then strain. I start drinking the tea two days before my period and continue until day two. The tea relaxes me, increases my calcium levels and reduces cramping. I often combine it with ginger tea.*

Acupuncture: *If I do get cramps, I just go and see myself for acupuncture, and while I'm getting it, I dream or read or create poems. Spending time doing what you find most relaxing is a fantastic tonic to add to your list!*

If you still need more help, try referring to Chapter 6 (the chapter on PMS). For example, chastetree berry, taken over time, can help to reduce period pain.

8

Menorrhagia (Excessive Blood Flow)

S ome women suffer from such heavy bleeding that they feel drained and lethargic from loss of blood. If left untreated, the heavy blood loss can lead to anemia and general weakening of the body from lack of vitamins and minerals.

Bleeding is considered severe if you soak through a pad or tampon in an hour or less.

Causes

Some functional causes of heavy bleeding include fibroids, cysts, tumors, anemia, thyroid problems and endometriosis. These functional causes should first be ruled out and addressed if they are found. However, the suggestions that follow will still be of aid, so read on.

Heavy bleeding can also be caused by imbalances of various organ systems in your body, especially the endocrine system, which includes the thyroid and the liver. When you nourish these organs and glands, your bleeding may be reduced to a normal flow.

Other causes of heavy bleeding include fragile blood vessels and circulatory problems, stress, vitamin and mineral deficiencies, especially deficiencies of calcium, iron and vitamins A and K.

Fortunately, these imbalances and deficiencies can be corrected using diet, herbs, vitamins and minerals.

Conventional Treatment

Most women who suffer from heavy bleeding are put on the birth control pill or told they need to have their uterus surgically removed. This surgery is not without risks. Certainly, without a uterus, a woman cannot conceive; her bone health may be at risk and her internal organs can prolapse. Some doctors recommend removing just the fibroid or endometrial tissue; however, these tissues may grow back if the underlying causes of the heavy bleeding are not corrected.

Foods that Heal

Eat from the Sea

Include seaweed in your daily diet. It's high in many minerals and vitamins that support bodily functions. Seaweed also supports the endocrine system, especially the thyroid glands. Try kelp, nori, dulse, hijike and kombu.

Eat Your Greens

Eat plenty of dark green leafy vegetables like kale, chard, broccoli, collard greens, mustard greens, beet greens and bok choy. They're loaded in iron and vitamin K, which help stop bleeding, and they contain other important vitamins and minerals. Eat them daily or drink them in juices.

Eat Whole Foods

Eat whole grains, legumes, seeds, nuts and high-quality vegetable protein to ensure high-quality nutrition. This will help to stop heavy bleeding.

Cut Out the Harmful Foods and Substances

Reduce or eliminate red meat, refined foods, excess salt, simple carbohydrates, sweets, alcohol, caffeine and junk food. These foods contribute to the organ imbalances that cause the heavy bleeding. Try to avoid aspirin, which can aggravate bleeding and thin the blood.

Herbs that Help

The Supreme Herb for Heavy Bleeding: Shepherd's Purse

This is an astringent herb that helps dry up excess fluids, so it is particularly useful for women who suffer from heavy bleeding. You can use it every half-hour until the bleeding has subsided, or you can start it several days before your period begins, to prevent heavy bleeding. Use fresh, not dried, shepherd's purse only, as an infused tea; or use it in a tincture made from the fresh herb.

Dosage: Take 30 to 40 drops of the tincture three to four times per day, or every half-hour on an empty stomach as needed. Or take three to four cups of the infused tea on an empty stomach. You can also start this regimen several days before your period begins and continue to follow it until heavy bleeding subsides.

Nettle

This herb is rich in iron and other valuable nutrients that can replace damaged or low iron stores. Nettle is an astringent herb that dries up bleeding.

Dosage: Take 40 to 150 drops three to four times per day on an empty stomach. In pill or tea form, take 2 to 5 grams three times per day on an empty stomach.

Cinnamon

Cinnamon is of great value in treating uterine bleeding. Some of my clients have had very good results using cinnamon with other astringent herbs. It is of special value because it makes unpleasant-tasting herbs palatable.

Dosage: Take 40 drops three to four times per day on an empty stomach. In pill form, take 2 to 4 grams per day. As a tea, infuse or decoct ½ to 1 tsp (2 mL to 4 mL) per cup (250 mL) of hot water three times per day on an empty stomach.

Yarrow

Yarrow, another astringent herb, is wonderful for stopping bleeding and is especially useful for excessive uterine bleeding or other bleeding from the reproductive tract. Herbalist Rosemary Gladstar recommends that you start taking it several days before your menstrual cycle begins to prevent heavy bleeding.

Dosage: Take 40 to 100 drops three times per day on an empty stomach. If in pill form, take 4 ½ grams per day. As a tea, drink an infusion of 1 to 2 tsp (4 mL to 10 mL) in one cup (250 mL) of water three times per day on an empty stomach.

Red Raspberry

Red raspberry leaf has been used for centuries for all kinds of women's health disorders. It is another astringent herb and is particularly useful for frequent or excessive bleeding.

Dosage: Take 40 drops three to four times per day on an empty stomach. For the tea, infuse 1 to 2 tsp (4 mL to 10 mL) in one cup (250 mL) of water and drink freely.

Liver Herbs: Dandelion Root, Boldo, Milk Thistle, Yellow Dock, Artichoke, Turmeric

These herbs help the liver to detoxify excess estrogen, breaking it down for excretion. Eliminating excess estrogen helps to correct hormonal imbalances that may lead to excess or prolonged bleeding (see Chapter 3).

Dosage: 40 drops of a tincture or liquid extract of one or more three times per day on an empty stomach.

Chastetree Berry

This herb balances estrogen and progesterone levels, thereby normalizing your menstrual cycle. Balanced hormones can reduce bleeding—even bleeding caused by fibroids, cysts and endometriosis. Use chastetree berry every day. If you're treating heavy bleeding, take it with liver herbs, astringents and licorice to strengthen your adrenal glands and balance your system.

Dosage: 3 to 6 grams of dried and ground berries, or 30 drops of the tincture, three times per day on an empty stomach. Chastetree berry is often standardized for 0.5 percent agnuside. If you are using a standardized tablet, take 175 to 225 mg daily; if a liquid extract, take 2 to 4 mL a day.

Energizing Iron

Since anemia is both a cause of heavy bleeding and a result of it, supplementing your diet with iron is vital if you are anemic. There are many forms of iron. Two of the best forms—*ferrous succinate* and *fumerate*—are easily absorbed and don't cause constipation. You can also take herbs rich in iron; for example, yellow dock, parsley, alfalfa, raspberry and nettle. To absorb the iron, take it with foods rich in vitamin C, or take vitamin C in supplement form. You can also try taking rosehip, a herb high in vitamin C. In addition to helping you absorb iron, vitamin C seems to help in its own right. When women with menorrhagia were given vitamin C with bioflavonoids, 88 percent of them improved. B vitamins also aid proper absorption and use of iron.

Dosage: Excess iron is linked to heart problems. So take iron in appropriate dosages only. Your need for iron is best determined by a blood test. The usual dosage for most menstruating women is 18 mg a day, but dosages vary widely, depending on your blood iron levels and stores. It is good to take iron with 1,000 mg of vitamin C and 50 mg of B complex every day with food.

Multivitamin and Mineral

It is also a very good idea to take a high-potency multivitamin and mineral to correct any underlying deficiencies.

THE ULTIMATE HEAVY BLEEDING FORMULAS

These three formulas are fantastic and work wonders. Though the teas may take a little time to prepare, they are well worth the effort. For a reminder on how to prepare a herbal tea, turn to page 36. For a simpler version, use the tinctures in Version Three.

Version One

For uterine bleeding, including the heavy bleeding of endometriosis, decoct 1 tsp (5 mL) each of the hard parts of agrimony, bayberry and cinnamon bark in three cups (750 mL) of water. Boil and then simmer the decoction. Remove from heat, add 1 tsp (5 mL) of nettle and cover for twenty minutes. Strain and drink a cupful every hour until the bleeding subsides.

Version Two

Another great herbal combination uses yarrow, shepherd's purse, nettles, red raspberry leaf and cinnamon bark. Decoct half a teaspoon (2 mL) of cinnamon bark in ½ cupful (125 ml) for forty minutes. Remove from heat. Infuse 1 teaspoon (5 mL) each of yarrow, nettle, raspberry leaf and shepherd's purse in 3 cups of water (750 ml). Mix the infusion and the decoction together. Drink a cupful every half-hour when bleeding is present. It can also be drunk, by the cupful, three times per day throughout the month to strengthen your system.

Version Three

Take 40 drops each (tinctures or liquid extracts) of shepherd's purse, yarrow and nettle three to four times per day on an empty stomach. Begin on day fourteen of your cycle or a few days before your period begins, depending on the severity of your symptoms. It can be used more frequently, as needed.

Finally an End to Heavy Bleeding

Some women take time to respond to treatments for heavy bleeding; others respond right away. I gave acupuncture to one woman as part of a treatment for heavy bleeding. She took yarrow four times per day on an empty stomach, beginning a few days before her period and continuing until day four. She also took a 225-mg standardized tablet of chastetree berry. Her heavy bleeding subsided immediately!

Not everyone responds this quickly, so stick to your program. You'll see results. Often the body needs time to balance itself and regain strength. Expect to wait three to six months for your system to correct itself, longer if your problem has been long-standing.

The Protocol for Heavy Bleeding

Follow the dietary suggestions given in this chapter. Be sure to include sea vegetables, like dulse, kelp and nori, and eat deep greens. Eat whole foods: whole grains, legumes, vegetables, fruit, raw seeds and nuts. Reduce red meat. Also reduce or eliminate refined foods, excess salt, aspirin, simple carbohydrates, sweets, alcohol, caffeine and junk food.

Take any one or a combination of shephard's purse, yarrow or nettle.

Shepherd's purse: *30 to 40 drops three to four times per day or every half-hour, as needed, on an empty stomach. You can begin this several days before your period starts and continue until heavy bleeding subsides. Take it more often if heavy bleeding persists.*

Yarrow: *40 to 100 drops three times per day on an empty stomach. For the pill, take 4½ grams per day on an empty stomach. As a tea, take an infusion of 1 to 2 tsp (4 to 10 mL) three times per day on an empty stomach.*

Nettle: *40 to 150 drops three to four times per day on an empty stomach. For the pill or tea forms, take 2 to 5 grams three times per day on an empty stomach.*

Multivitamin and mineral: *Take a high-potency multivitamin and mineral with your food to supply the B vitamins, vitamin C and iron. You may need additional iron.*

This may be all you need to bring your body into balance. However, you may also want to consider some additional support:

Try any one of the three fantastic Ultimate Heavy Bleeding Formulas listed above and/or:

Chastetree berry: *3 to 6 grams of the dried and ground berries three times a day, of the tincture 30 drops three times a day. Chastetree berry is often standardized for 0.5 percent agnuside. If you are using a standardized tablet, take 175 mg to 225 mg daily; if a liquid extract, take 2 to 4 mL a day.*

Liver herbs: *Add a combination of liver herbs, like artichoke, boldo, dandelion root, yellow dock and milk thistle to your daily regime: 40 drops of one or each three times per day on an empty stomach.*

9

Amenorrhea (Absence of Periods)

S ome women experience a total or partial lack of their menstrual cycles. Their periods just stop. A stoppage of three months or more is considered amenorrhea.

Causes

There can be numerous causes for this stoppage. Today, the most common causes of lack of menstruation are improper diet, anorexia or bulimia, or overly rigorous exercise. With all the pressure for women to look skinny in today's world, many women are simply not getting the nutrition they need, especially good quality protein and good fats. The result is pallor, fatigue, poor health and lack of menstruation. In the United States, amenorrhea occurs in 1.8 to 3 percent of women.

Other causes of amenorrhea include tumors, emotional stress and trauma, hormonal imbalances, obesity and the birth control pill. The pill is one of the worst culprits. Many women go off the pill in the hopes of re-establishing their normal menstrual cycle, and they can wait months or even years for its return. Some women do not get any periods at all for some time after being on the pill.[1] And so some women are unable to conceive after they stop taking the pill, because they don't ovulate right away.

It's always a good idea to see a practitioner to rule out any serious underlying causes for the lack of menstruation. Amenorrhea is often caused by disorders of the vagina, uterus, ovaries, pituitary gland, central nervous system, thyroid gland and hypothalamus and these causes should be looked into.

Conventional Treatment

Conventional medicine primarily deals with lack of menstruation by placing women on hormone therapy, but hormone therapy is not without risks. Chemical hormones are believed to increase a woman's risk of cancer—especially breast cancer—and heart disease. Other conventional treatments include surgical removal of tumors; dopamine agonist therapy to reduce prolactin secretion; and anti-estrogen therapies. Prolactin-reducing drugs—for example, Bromocriptine—can have side effects such as severe nausea, vomiting and dizziness.[2] Anti-estrogen drugs—for example, Tamoxifen—also have side effects. They can cause nausea, vomiting, hot flashes, swollen ankles, skin rashes and liver damage.[3]

But there are other fantastic choices for women who don't have periods. Herbs, vitamins and nutrition can often correct or re-establish a normal cycle.

Foods that Heal

Since malnutrition is one of the most frequent causes of amenorrhea, the very first thing to do is improve your diet and make sure you're getting a full range of vitamins, minerals, fats, protein and fiber. Your diet should include whole foods, with ample essential fatty acids, such as flaxseed oil and other healthy fats. Take 1 to 2 tbsp (15 mL to 25 mL) of flaxseed oil daily. Eat lots of vegetables, seeds, nuts, legumes, fruits, seaweeds and whole grains frequently.

What to Eat

It's really simple. A diet that is rich in nutrients includes these wonderful foods:

- Four to nine servings of whole grains a day.
- Six to eight servings, or more, of vegetables, including at least one dark green vegetable such as chard, kale, collard greens, broccoli, spinach, beet greens and bok choy.
- Yellow, orange, white and red vegetables should also be included frequently.
- Sprouts—try broccoli, radish, alfalfa, mung bean and red clover sprouts. They are a powerhouse of nutrition. Use them in sandwiches and salads; eat them as a snack.
- One to three servings a day or more of legumes: soy, lentils, black beans, mung beans, kidney beans, romano beans, pinto beans and chickpeas, etc. Try hummus, soy burgers, tofu dogs, tofu, soy milk, soy ice cream, lentil soup, bean chili, bean soup, Jamaican beans and rice dishes, bean salads, Indian dal, bean dips and Ethiopian wats (bean stews) The international world of cuisine has much to offer in this food group.
- Raw unsalted seeds and nuts: almonds, hazelnuts, pumpkin seeds, sesame seeds, flaxseeds and sunflower seeds. Carry these around for quick and easy snacks.
- Two to three servings, or more, of fruit a day. Try all the raw fruits: apples, oranges, grapefruit, mangos, kiwifruit, berries, pomegranate, pears, plums, peaches, pineapple and mangosteen, etc. Try baked fruits, fruit purees, fruit salads, fruit muffins and fruit cakes made with whole grain flour and sweetened with fruit.

Reduce or avoid caffeine, chocolate, alcohol and refined carbohydrates: they aggravate amenorrhea (and are empty foods without adequate nutritional value).

If you're underweight, I encourage you to achieve healthy weight gain. If you're overweight, I encourage you to achieve healthy weight loss. Both too much and too little weight are causes of amenorrhea. (For advice on healthy weight, turn to Chapters 5 and 16.)

Foods for Bone Health

Foods that support bone health are important, since women who don't have periods are at risk for bone problems. Poor nutrition can lead to a lack of, or imbalance of, hormones, especially estrogen and progesterone, which can cause poor bones. Eat dark leafy greens, like kale, chard and bok choy; eat soy foods; eat sea vegetables, like dulse, kelp and nori; eat whole grains and legumes. All these foods will support bone health.

Herbs that Help

Many herbs are known as *emmenagogues*: herbs that bring on menstrual flow. Any of them are good choices and are often combined together. So feel free to experiment.

Black Cohosh and Blue Cohosh

Black cohosh and blue cohosh are emmenagogues that can be used to bring on periods. Blue cohosh traditionally has been more frequently used for this purpose. Traditional herbalists consider blue cohosh as one of the most powerful choices. Often blue and black cohosh are combined with dong quai, cramp bark and ginger.

Dosage: 40 drops of either one, or both, three to four times per day on an empty stomach.

Mugwort, Myrrh and Motherwort

These three herbs are also emmenagogues. Motherwort helps relax the nerves and can help when the period stopped because of nervous tension. If the menstrual cycle has been absent for a long time, mugwort is a good choice; many traditional herbalists would try mugwort first. Feel free to try any of them, or combine them.

Dosages
- Mugwort: 20 to 40 drops three times per day on an empty stomach. As a tea, use 3 to 9 grams per cup, three times per day on an empty stomach.

- Myrrh: 40 to 80 drops three times per day on an empty stomach.
- Motherwort: 40 drops three to four times per day on an empty stomach. As a pill, 4½ grams on an empty stomach.

Chastetree Berry

Hormonal imbalance can stop the period; chastetree berry can balance hormones. It is of particular value for women who lack enough progesterone or whose pituitary or hypothalamus need modulating. It can also reduce excess prolactin levels (too much prolactin is another cause of amenorrhea).[4] As well, chastetree berry can correct periods made irregular or absent by the birth control pill.

Dosage: The usual dosage of chastetree berry is 3 to 6 grams of the dried and ground berries three times a day, of the tincture 30 drops three times a day. Chastetree berry is often standardized for 0.5 percent agnuside. If you are using a standardized tablet, take 175 to 225 mg daily; if a liquid extract, take half a teaspoon (2 mL) a day.

Red Clover, Soy, Flaxseeds and Other Phytoestrogens

Many herbs/foods are considered to be phytoestrogenic, which means they can help balance your body's own estrogen level, raising it if it is too low and lowering it if it is too high.[5] (See Soy in Chapter 5.) This action can be useful in treating amenorrhea, since it supports the menstrual cycle and corrects underlying imbalances. Phytoestrogenic herbs include red clover, alfalfa, flaxseed, hops and soy. You can also eat flaxseed, alfalfa and red clover sprouts. You can take the herbs in pills or tinctures. Many formulas combine several of these herbs. Feel free to experiment: they are all good choices.

Dosages

- Alfalfa: Eat alfalfa sprouts liberally in your diet, or take 500 to 1,000 mg in pill form.
- Flaxseeds: Eat 1 to 4 tablespoons (15 mL to 60 mL) of flaxseeds each day.
- Hops: 40 drops of the tincture three to four times a day on an empty stomach.
- Soy: Enjoy soy in your diet freely.
- Red clover: Enjoy the sprouts in your salads and sandwiches, or drink an infusion of 2 to 3 tsp (10 mL to 15 mL) per cup (250 mL) of water three times a day. Or you can take 40 to 80 drops of the tincture three times a day. You can also take 2 to 4 grams in pill form each day.

Red Raspberry Leaf and Nettle

Both red raspberry leaf and nettle are often used in suppressed menstruation to strengthen the system and for their nutritive properties.

Dosages

- Red Raspberry: 40 drops three to four times per day on an empty stomach. For the tea, infuse 1 to 2 tsp (4 mL to 10 mL) in one cup (250 mL) of water and drink freely.
- Nettle: 40 to 150 drops three to four times per day on an empty stomach. For pill or tea forms, take 2 to 5 grams three times per day on an empty stomach.

Herbs for Stress: Skullcap, Passionflower, Valerian, Linden, Ginseng, Licorice, Kava

If lack of periods is caused by stress, then anti-stress herbs, like skullcap, kava—if available—passionflower, valerian and linden can be useful. Though all of these herbs are great choices for relieving stress and inducing sleep, if your stress is accompanied by anxiety, then kava, passionflower and valerian may be the best choices. Valerian is also a great choice if your stress causes insomnia. Herbs that support the adrenal glands (the glands that help your body deal with stress) such as ginseng and licorice are also very useful.

Dosages

- Skullcap: 40 to 80 drops of the tincture or 3 grams of the pill three times a day on an empty stomach. You can also drink an infusion of 1 to 2 tsps (4 mL to 10 mL) three times a day on an empty stomach. .
- Kava: 45 to 70 mg of kavalactones (a marker for active ingredient in kava) three times a day.
- Passionflower: 40 drops three or four times per day, or as needed, on an empty stomach. If you prefer pills, take 2 grams three to four times a day.
- Valerian: 150 to 300 mg (0.8 percent valeric acid) 30 minutes before bed, or 40 drops three to four times a day.
- Linden: 20 to 40 drops three times a day on an empty stomach. If taking in tea form, infuse 1 tsp (4 mL) per cup (250 mL) of water and enjoy it three times a day.
- Ginseng: 1 to 9 grams a day.
- Licorice: If using the powder, take 1 to 2 grams three times a day; if using the fluid extract (1:1), take ½ to 1 tsp (2 mL to 4 mL) three times a day; if using the solid dry powdered extract (4:1), take 250 to 500 mg three times a day.

Pennyroyal

Pennyroyal is often used externally as an oil (do not use the oil internally) or in a herbal bath to help bring on absent periods. This herb is an emmenagogue and has a special affinity for the female reproductive organs. Rub a few drops, or more, onto the abdomen, or use a carrier oil like almond oil, or put into a bath.

Natural Progesterone Cream

Natural progesterone cream can also be of use in re-establishing normal menstruation, if progesterone is low as determined by blood tests. This cream should be used under supervision, as dosage must be determined based on each individual.

Vitamins, Minerals and Other Useful Supplements

B6

Many women with absent periods have been found to have B6 deficiencies.[5]

Dosage: 50 mg three times per day with food. Or you can take it as a B-complex, 50 mg three times per day with food.

Zinc

Women with absent periods tend to be deficient in zinc.[5] It is believed to be a cause of anorexia, which can lead to amenorrhea. Zinc is involved in reproductive health.

Dosage: 25 to 50 mg, balanced with 2 to 3 mg of copper, three times per day with food.

Iron

Women who have not been eating well are often low in iron.

Dosage: If a blood test determines you are low in iron, take as directed by a health-care professional.

Calcium, Magnesium and Other Bone Nutrients

Women with prolonged amenorrhea are at serious risk for developing bone problems. The risk increases because there is a decrease in the rate of absorption of calcium in women who are estrogen deficient.[6] So women who are not menstruating need to take in more calcium and other bone nutrients.

Dosage: Many health food stores have formulas designed specifically to build your bones. They contain magnesium, manganese, zinc, copper, boron and vitamins K, D, C and B vitamins. Make sure the formula you buy contains at least 1,200 to 1,500 mg of calcium; 600 mg of magnesium; 1,000 IU of vitamin D; and 25 mg of zinc. These formulas should be taken once per day with food. You can also try ipriflavone. This nutrient helps maintain bone mass and, when combined with calcium, helps increase it.[7]

Multivitamin and Mineral Complex

Missed or stopped periods are often caused by a lack of nutrition, so it's a good idea to take a high-quality, high-potency multivitamin and mineral formula to help establish any nutrients that may be missing from your diet. I often suggest that clients use more than one a day for a while.

The Mind Connection

Many natural health practitioners suggest that a woman try to remember when her periods used to come and to think of them as still coming at that time. This helps re-establish a normal cycle. Women are also encouraged to hang around with women who are menstruating; this can too help bring on menstruation too. Not only have I seen this work in my practice, but it has also been demonstrated in studies. Menstruating women secrete pheromones that can stimulate menstruation in other women.

Finally, an End to Amenorrhea

It's a good idea to work with a practitioner to find out why you're not menstruating and to work with the practitioner. It takes time to re-establish a normal menstrual cycle, so do not expect quick results. But with the right diagnosis and careful attention to a comprehensive program, amenorrhea can be overcome.

The Protocol for Amenorrhea

Follow the dietary suggestions outlined in this chapter so you can establish a normal, healthy weight. Eat 1 to 2 tablespoons (15 mL to 30 mL) of flaxseed oil daily.

Blue or black cohosh: *40 drops of one, or of each, three times per day on an empty stomach.*

Motherwort: *40 drops three times per day on an empty stomach.*

Valerian: *40 drops three times per day on an empty stomach. For stress.*

Alfalfa: *40 drops three times per day on an empty stomach. For extra nutrition.*

Nettle: *40 drops three times per day on an empty stomach. For extra nutrition.*

Multivitamin: *Take a high potency multivitamin/mineral compound.*

B-complex: *Take 50 mg of B6 three times per day with food. Or take 50 mg of a B-complex three times per day with food.*

Bone Formula: *1,200 to 1,500 mg, or more, of calcium; 600 mg of magnesium, 1,000 IU of vitamin D and 25 mg of zinc, all with food.*

This may be all you need to bring your body back into balance. However, you may also want to consider some additional support:

Chastetree berry: *3 to 6 grams of the dried and ground berries three times a day; of the tincture, 30 drops three times a day. Chastetree berry is often standardized for 0.5 percent agnuside. If you are using a standardized tablet, take 175 to 225 mg daily; if a liquid extract, take ½ teaspoon (2 mL) a day.*

If still further help is needed, try any of the other suggestions given in this chapter.

10

Preventing and Treating Fibrocystic
Breast Disease

A s many as 40 percent of all women get fibrocystic breast disease (FBD). That's how common it is. Many sufferers never find relief for this painful condition. But FBD is treatable; in fact, the problem can be completely reversed using supplements and simple, effective dietary and lifestyle changes and some supplements.

What Is FBD?

FBD is characterized by painful lumps in the breasts and is usually related to PMS. At one time, it was thought that women who had FBD were more likely to develop breast cancer. They're not, although one cause of fibrocystic breast disease, iodine deficiency, may be linked to breast cancer. Excess estrogen could be another link. Both conditions can be corrected.

Causes

There are many causes of fibrocystic breast disease. The most common is probably too much estrogen in the body. Excess estrogen can come from eating red meat and dairy foods—which are high in estrogen—or taking birth control pills, or from environmental sources such as plastics. Other causes include stress, candida, poor diet, sluggish liver and caffeine.

Caffeine is a real culprit. In one study, women eliminated caffeine altogether, and 97.5 percent of them improved. Of the women who cut caffeine way down, 75 percent improved.[1] Coffee, tea, cola, chocolate and other foods high in caffeine all contain methylxanthine, which may cause fibrocystic breast disease in women who are sensitive to methylxanthine. You may want to try dandelion root tea to help you make the switch from caffeine: it tastes a little like coffee, and it detoxifies the liver, which helps get rid of excess estrogen.

Foods that Heal

Fiber

An important dietary change that can help women recover from FBD is to switch to a high-fiber diet, preferably one that is primarily vegetarian. Most animal foods are too high in estrogen, or cause estrogen levels to go up in the body, which causes the problem, but also studies have linked a diet low in fiber to FBD and cancer. Finally, a diet low in fiber contributes to constipation, and women who have fewer than three bowel movements a week are far more likely to suffer from

FBD than women who have daily bowel movements. This connection seems to be due to the bad bacterial flora in the large intestine that make toxic substances and/or allow toxic substances to be reabsorbed. A lack of dietary fiber encourages improper bacterial flora. These bad bacteria make an enzyme called glucoronidase that frees estrogen from the glucoronic acid that attaches to it in order to escort it out of the body: so estrogen increases.

Interestingly, dietary fiber is associated with a decreased risk of breast disease and breast cancer. This may be because excess estrogen is excreted. Women who eat a vegetarian diet excrete two to three times more estrogen than women who eat meat, and they have 55 percent less unbound estrogen in their blood.

Reduce or Eliminate Dairy Products

It is important that you cut out all dairy products, since they can raise estrogen levels, which, in turn, can cause FBD. They can also encourage bad bacterial growth, and they have no fiber, so your body does not properly eliminate waste and toxins further build up, leading to FBD.

Iodine: Eat from the Sea

Clinical studies have shown that people with FBD can recover using iodine therapy. Iodine therapy can also reduce serum prolactin levels, breast lumps and breast tenderness. Most people do not get enough iodine in their diets. Kelp, dulse, nori and other sea vegetables provide a good source of iodine and can be used in soups, salads, stews, pastas or whatever you like, or they can be taken in convenient tablet form. Why not make the need for iodine the excuse you've been looking for to visit the sea or ocean? Even walking beside the ocean can increase your iodine levels. Going for a swim is even better. Taking an iodine supplement may support an underactive thyroid, which is also linked to FBD.

Dosage: Take 70 to 90 mcg of caseinate or liquid iodine for each kilogram of body weight once a day.

Reduce Stress

It is vitally important that some method be used to reduce stress in women with FBD. Women can completely reverse FBD by eliminating stress and taking the proper supplements. Try meditation. Or try acupuncture: it can rebalance your body and help you relax.

Herbs and Supplements that Help

B vitamins

A healthy liver is key to treating FBD: it is the liver's job to clear excess estrogen from your body. Your liver binds estrogen to glucoronic acid, then excretes it in the bile. This process requires B6, folic acid and the other B vitamins. Any deficiency in any of the B vitamins can cause FBD. Any liver disease (for example, a toxic liver) and any environmental pollution may interfere with normal liver function, causing a buildup of excess estrogen, which can cause FBD.

Dosage: 100 to 200 mg of vitamin B6 per day with food. Take 50 mg at a time. Take B6 throughout your menstrual cycle and in conjunction with a B-complex to relieve breast pain.

Liver Herbs

Milk thistle, dandelion root, yellow dock and Oregon grape root also are good for supporting the liver.

Dosage: 40 drops of one or more of these herbs, three to four times per day, half an hour before each meal.

Essential Fatty Acids

People with FBD tend to have abnormal prolactin levels. Take evening primrose oil, borage oil or flaxseed oil to normalize prolactin levels. Several studies have found that taking evening primrose oil provides relief.[2]

Dosage: 1 to 2 tablespoons (15 mL to 30 mL) of evening primrose oil, borage oil or flaxseed oil a day. I prefer using flaxseed oil, as it is richer in omega 3s, and is less inflammatory than omega 6s.

Wild Yam Cream and Progesterone Cream

One approach to treating FBD is getting very good results: using natural, safe creams to adjust the hormone balance by increasing progesterone levels. In a study of patients with FBD, Dr. Mauvais-Jarvis found decreased progesterone to estrogen levels. In 95 percent of these patients, a natural progesterone cream rubbed into the breasts relieved breast pain. Wild yam cream contains components that have similar properties to progesterone. Either wild yam or natural progesterone cream can be used. It is usually made for individuals and should come with specific advice about use.

Chastetree Berry

The herb chastetree berry works by balancing estrogen and progesterone levels in your body, so it's ideal for treating FBD. Chastetree berry usually takes a minimum of three months to have an effect; long-term results are usually obtained after one full year of continual use.

Dosage: 3 to 6 grams of the dried and ground berries three times a day; of the tincture, 30 drops three times a day. Chastetree berry is often standardized for 0.5 percent agnuside. If you are using a standardized tablet, take 175 to 225 mg daily; if using a liquid extract, take ½ teaspoon (2 mL) a day.

Vitamin E

Several double-blind studies have shown vitamin E to be very useful in treating FBD. Vitamin E works on patients with FBD by normalizing circulating hormones. It has been shown to normalize the elevated levels of pituitary hormones FSH and LH that are often found in people with FBD.

Dosage: 600 IU of vitamin E per day with food.

Vitamin A

Another abnormality that shows up in women with FBD is low levels of vitamin A. Supplementing with very high levels of vitamin A can reduce or completely eliminate FBD. Such high levels of vitamin A are not safe for long-term use: be careful if you undertake this therapy. Use only under supervision.

Probiotics

Lactobacilus acidophilus can help women with FBD: acidophilus promotes the excretion of estrogen.

Dosage: Take 2 billion to 20 billion live cultures a day on an empty stomach. The higher dosages are used by some people and are usually taken only for two weeks.

Further Help

Other key nutrients for treating FBD include herbs that support your immune system—for example, shiitake, maitake and reishi mushrooms; antioxidants, for example, vitamin C and beta-carotene; fat-dissolving nutrients, for example, lecithin; and herbs that shrink masses, for example, pau d'arco. Herbs that support the lymph system, for example, red root, echinacea and cleavers, can also help.

Dosages

- Shiitake: 40 to 80 drops of the tincture daily. If you are using the pill, take 400 mg to 2 grams per day on an empty stomach.
- Maitake: 3 to 7 grams per day.
- Reishi: 3 grams three times per day.
- Vitamin C: 500 to 1,000 mg three times per day with food.
- Beta-carotene: 50,000 to 300,000 IU per day.
- Lecithin: 1200 mg before each meal.
- Pau d'arco: 3 to 4 cups (750 mL to 1 L) per day as a decoction, on an empty stomach.
- Red root, echinacea and cleavers: 40 drops of one or each, three to four times per day, on an empty stomach.

Topical Help

It is equally important to treat this problem topically. Try using castor oil packs on the breasts for an hour or more four times a week. Castor oil packs alleviate pain and inflammation, and can be used for detoxifying purposes. See page 93 for how to make them. Other useful topical agents include green clay packs for detoxifying (use four times a week) and poke root (apply daily). Poke root has been used traditionally for years to reduce all kinds of breast lumps, including cancer. Or try acupuncture, which can rebalance the body and shrink lumps.

Finally, an End to FBD

With a little time and effort you will soon reduce those painful lumps—and PMS as well—while simultaneously reducing your risk for breast cancer.

The Protocol for FBD

Follow the dietary guidelines given in this chapter: eat a high-fiber diet, rich in sea vegetables and low in animal products, and reduce or eliminate caffeine. Reduce your level of stress; try acupuncture to break up masses and lumps.

Iodine: *70 to 90 mcg of iodine (caseinate or liquid iodine) per kilogram of body weight a day. Eat sea vegetables like nori, kelp and dulse.*

Flaxseed oil or evening primose oil: *1 to 2 tbsp (15 mL to 30 mL) a day.*

B6 along with a B-complex: *50 mg of B6 and/or 50 mg of a B complex three times per day with each meal.*

Liver herbs: *Milk thistle, dandelion root, yellow dock and Oregon grape root: 40 drops of one or each, three times per day on an empty stomach.*

Vitamin E: *600 IU per day with food.*

Probiotics: *Take 2 billion to 20 billion live cultures a day on an empty stomach. The higher dosages are used by some people and are usually taken only for two weeks.*

Chastetree Berry: *For hormone balance, take 3 to 6 grams of the dried and ground berries three times a day; of the tincture, 30 drops three times a day. Chastetree berry is often standardized for 0.5 percent agnuside. If you are using a standardized tablet, take 175 to 225 mg daily; if a liquid extract, take ½ tsp (2 mL) a day.*

This may be all you need to bring your body back into balance. However, you may also want to consider some additional support:

Topical Support

Use a topical application of castor oil or green clay four times per week, all through the month. Try poke root, applied topically, daily.

Immune System Support

Try using shiitake, maitake and reishi mushrooms.

- *Shiitake: 40 to 80 drops of the tincture daily. If you are taking the pill, use 400 mg to 2 grams per day on an empty stomach.*
- *Maitake: 3 to 7 grams per day.*
- *Reishi: 3 grams three times per day.*

Antioxidants

Take 500 to 1,000 mg of vitamin C three times per day with food, and 50,000 to 300,000 IU of beta-carotene daily.

Fat-Dissolving Nutrient

Take 1,200 mg of lecithin before each meal.

Mass-Shrinking Herb

Drink a decoction of pau d'arco three to four times per day on an empty stomach.

Lymph-Supporting Herbs

Use red root, echinacea and cleavers: 40 drops of one or each, three to four times per day on an empty stomach.

11

Eliminating Ovarian Cysts and Uterine Fibroids

M any women will have both ovarian cysts and uterine fibriods. Both are also related to hormones being out of balance. As with PMS, if you correct your hormone imbalance, you will greatly reduce the problems.

Symptoms

Some women have no symptoms, but most will experience pain, excessive menstrual bleeding, painful periods and pain in the pelvic region. Other symptoms include a distended abdomen, which can mirror the early stages of pregnancy.

What Is a Cyst?

An ovarian cyst is a semisolid material that develops in the ovarian tissue. Cysts often occur when follicles fail to rupture or release the egg during the normal cycle; these follicles fill with fluid, become semisolid and develop into little sacs called ovarian cysts. Cysts can also appear during the formation of the corpus luteum in the hormone cycle.

What Is a Fibroid?

Uterine fibroids are noncancerous tumors, generally solid, that occur in the uterus and can range in size from tiny, 1 cm, to very large, the size of a grapefruit. There can be just one or many.

Causes

Cysts and fibroids seem to develop in the presence of estrogen. Sometimes the liver is not able to break down and excrete excess estrogen. Oral contraceptives, pregnancy and estrogen treatments all stimulate the growth of fibroids. Constipation and toxin buildup can lead to fibroids and cysts. Fortunately, both cysts and fibroids respond extremely well to natural treatments and can often be totally eliminated without drugs or surgery.

Foods that Heal

The underlying cause of ovarian cysts and uterine fibroids is an elevated level of estrogen, which is also a cause of PMS, so turn to Chapter 5 for the ultimate diet to follow. This diet focuses on cleansing foods and foods that don't raise estrogen. Eat whole grains, fruits, vegetables, seeds, legumes and raw nuts. Eat lots of dark green vegetables. These foods are all high in fiber, which reduces excess estrogen in your body and prevents constipation and toxin buildup, both of which cause cysts and fibroids. Consume essential fatty acids—flaxseed oil or hemp seed oil—and focus on foods that are high in antioxidants—vegetables, fruits, raw nuts, raw seeds, whole grains and legumes—as they can help detoxify estrogen. Eat foods high in sulfur-containing amino acids, for example, garlic, onions and beans.

Reduce or eliminate your intake of dairy products, eggs, red meat, sugar, white flour, refined foods, caffeine, chocolate, black and green teas and "bad" fat, as they can increase estrogen. Avoid storing foods in, or eating foods from, plastic containers, as this has been shown to increase estrogen in the body.

Herbs and Supplements that Help

The natural way of treating cysts and fibriods aims to detoxify the body, especially the liver; shrink growths; decrease inflammation in the pelvis; promote lymph drainage; and balance hormones. The liver is the main way that excess estrogen is detoxified from the body. Since cysts and fibroids are sensitive to estrogen, it is important to detoxify the liver.

Vitamin C

A good liver-cleansing solution includes vitamin C—it raises glutathione in the liver, which helps the liver detoxify.

Dosage: Try 1 to 5 grams or more a day of buffered vitamin C with food. Some women use more.

SAMe

SAMe is great for detoxifying the liver. It increases sulfur compounds, for example, glutathione, which are extremely good for detoxifying the liver. SAMe is also a lipotropic factor, a substance that removes excess fat from the liver, which helps the liver function better. SAMe is great for getting rid of excess estrogen.

Dosage: 400 to 1,500 mg a day in divided dosages. Start slowly, and build up the dosage biweekly. Don't use with other SSRIs or herbs that increase serotonin without supervision.

Detoxifying Herbs

Milk thistle, dandelion root, black radish, artichoke, burdock, yellow dock, wild yam, nettle and Oregon grape root are all excellent herbs that help to detoxify.

Dosage: Choose one or more from the list and take 40 drops of each three times per day on an empty stomach.

Turmeric

Turmeric is a wonderful and safe anti-inflammatory herb, and it is great for the liver.

Dosage: 40 drops three times per day on an empty stomach or 1 to 4 grams of the powdered root.

Lymph-Draining Herbs

Red root, echinacea and cleavers all support your lymph system and help it drain properly. Good drainage is an important aspect of treating cysts and fibroids.

Dosage: Choose one or two from the above list, and take 30 to 40 drops of each three times per day on an empty stomach.

Growth-Shrinking Herbs

Chaparral, shiitake mushrooms, reishi mushrooms and pau d'arco all naturally and safely encourage growths to shrink and disappear.

Dosage: Choose one or two of these herbs and take 40 drops of each three times per day on an empty stomach.

Essiac

This old herbal formula, a safe and reliable detoxifier for the body, is available in health food stores. It contains herbs that detoxify the body and is used for everything from fibroids and cysts to cancer.

Dosage: Follow the directions on the box.

Chastetree Berry

Chastetree berry reduces excess estrogen in the body and balances hormones. (See page 38 for detailed information of how chastetree berry works to balance hormones.)

Dosage: 3 to 6 grams of the dried and ground berries three times a day; of the tincture, 30 drops three times a day. Chastetree berry is often standardized for 0.5 percent agnuside. If you are using a standardized tablet, take 175 to 225 mg daily; if a liquid extract, take ½ teaspoon (2 mL) a day.

Wild Yam, Natural Progesterone

Wild yam cream and natural progesterone cream are also used for balancing hormones. Both increase levels of progesterone in the body and should be taken under the supervision of a trained health-care practitioner.

Phtyoestrogens

These herbs help balance elevated estrogen by stealing receptor sites from your body's more potent estrogen[1] and binding a weaker, safer kind of estrogen to them.[2] Phtyoestrogens include herbs like red clover, soy, fennel, licorice and alfalfa.

Dosages: All, except soy, should be taken on an empty stomach.

- Red clover: Drink an infusion of 2 to 3 tsp (10 mL to 15 mL) per cup (250 mL) of water one to three times a day. If you prefer, you can take anywhere from 40 to 80 drops of the tincture three times a day, or 2 to 4 grams in pill form each day.
- Soy: Enjoy soy in your diet freely.
- Fennel: 40 to 80 drops of the tincture three times a day.
- Licorice: If you use the powder, take 1 to 2 grams three times a day; if you use the fluid extract (1:1), take ½ to 1 tsp (2 mL to 4 mL) three times a day; if you use the solid dry powdered extract (4:1), take 250 to 500 mg three times a day.
- Alfalfa: 500 to 1,000 mg in pill form.

Herbs That Are Helpful in Shrinking Growths

Traditional herbs like motherwort, blue cohosh, black cohosh, red raspberry, blue vervain and lady's mantle are helpful in shrinking uterine fibroids and ovarian cysts. Many of these herbs offer additional support: Red raspberry tones and supports the female reproductive system. The cohoshes and motherwort help move blockages that can cause growths. Lady's mantle helps stop the excess bleeding that can accompany ovarian cysts and uterine fibroids. Blue vervain can help clear liver congestion.

Dosages

- Motherwort: 40 drops three to four times per day on an empty stomach. In pill form, take 4½ grams per day on an empty stomach.
- Blue cohosh: 40 drops three to four times per day on an empty stomach.
- Black cohosh: 40 drops three to four times per day on an empty stomach.
- Red raspberry: 40 drops three to four times per day on an empty stomach. For the tea, infuse 1 to 2 tsp (5 mL to 10 mL) in 1 cup (250 mL) of water and drink freely one to three cups a day.
- Blue vervain: 30 drops three times per day on an empty stomach, or infuse 1 teaspoon (5 mL) in 1 cup (250 mL) of water and drink three times a day on an empty stomach.
- Lady's mantle: Make an infusion of 2 tsp (10 mL) of the herb per 1 cup (250 mL) of water, and drink three cup per day on an empty stomach.

Other Useful Nutrients

Antioxidants eliminate excess estrogen from the body. Beta-carotene and selenium repair reproductive tissue and encourage cysts to disappear, while vitamin E regulates hormones and encourages healing of the reproductive tissues. Lipotrophic factors—choline and inositol—help detoxify and eliminate waste and fat from your liver, and a good multivitamin and mineral combination helps ensure you have all the nutrients you need for proper healing.

Dosages

- Beta-carotene: 50,000 IU per day with food.
- Selenium: 200 mcg per day with food.
- Vitamin E: 400 to 800 IU per day with food.
- Multivitamin and mineral: 1 per day with food.
- Lipotrophic factors: 1,000 mg of choline and inositol per day with food.

Vaginal Bolus

A vaginal bolus is an insert the size of your baby finger made up of herbs in a solid carrier that melts when inserted. Insert one five nights in a row, then rest for two nights; repeat this pattern for several weeks. I particularly love this adaptation of a traditional formula that herbalist Rosemary Gladstar, author of *Herbal Healing for Women,* gives. It's designed to get rid of uterine fibroids and ovarian cysts. I use it frequently in the clinic and get excellent results. You'll need coconut oil and herbs. Look for the herbs in the loose herb section of health food stores. Make as much of the herb mixture as you want and store it. Mix the herbs in these ratios:

- 1 part yellow dock root powder
- 1 part chaparral leaf powder
- 1 part goldenseal powder
- 3 parts slippery elm powder
- 1 part witch hazel bark powder
- ½ part black walnut hull powder
- 1 to 2 drops essential oil of myrrh and or tea tree oil

Melt 1 cup (250 mL) of solidified coconut oil on low heat. Remove from heat and mix in enough of the powdered herbs to make a thick paste. Add the oil of myrrh and or tea tree oil. Roll into boluses—about the size and shape of your little finger. Be careful not to burn yourself. Allow to cool. (The boluses will harden.) Insert the bolus far into the vagina. Wear a liner for the melting herb residue, and douche with 3 drops of grapefruit seed extract in distilled water every few days to remove residue. Store the boluses in a jar in the fridge. This remedy will help shrink growths like cysts and fibroids; it will dry up excessive bleeding; it will also prevent infection and provide relief from painful inflammation and irritation. It is totally safe and often provides quick relief.

Topical Applications

Poke Root

Use poke root externally in tincture form. I have seen this herb work wonders for breaking up congestion and shrinking growths.

Dosage: Apply a few drops to affected area and leave on overnight. Repeat five days a week, then rest for a day or two to give your body a chance to recover from detoxifying.

Castor Oil Packs

This old-time remedy has been used successfully by countless people to detoxify and achieve better health. Castor oil is a powerful detoxifier that can help the body shrink growths and break up stagnation and congestion.

Dosage: Warm castor oil and place it on the whole lower abdomen. Cover the liver area, too. According to tradition, cover with a red flannel and a hot water bottle. Leave on for one hour or more. Repeat for five days in a row, then rest for two. Repeat for several weeks, or months if needed.

Clay Packs

Try using green clay topically. Green clay has a strong ability to draw things out of the body and can reduce stagnation and congestion by increasing blood circulation to an area. It also breaks up cysts and fibroids.

Dosage: First rub a few drops of olive oil on your abdomen, then apply ½ to 1 cup (125 mL to 250 mL) of clay—green is best—mixed with enough water to get a thick paste. Cover with a piece of gauze. Leave on for one to two hours or overnight.

Needles to the Rescue

Acupuncture is excellent: it helps detoxify the liver, break up stagnation and congestion, rebalance the body and shrink cysts and fibroids.

Hot and Cold Baths

Try an old hydrotherapy remedy: the sitz bath. The sitz bath helps remove stagnation and congestion by increasing blood flow to an area. It also helps break up cysts and fibroids. You'll need two containers or buckets large enough for you to sit in. Fill one with the hottest water you can stand—don't burn yourself—and one with the coldest water you can stand. Start by sitting in the hot one for a few minutes, then switch to the cold one and sit in it for a minute or two. Go back and forth four times, finishing with the cold one. Do this for five days in a row, then rest for two. Repeat for several weeks, or even months if needed.

Finally, an End to Cysts and Fibroids

You'll be pleasantly surprised to see that, with a little time and effort, hormones can be brought into balance, and most cysts and fibroids can be eliminated safely and without surgery.

The Protocol for Cysts and Fibroids

Eat a cleansing diet. Turn to Chapter 5 for details on the perfect hormone-balancing diet. Focus on whole foods that are high in fiber and antioxidants—vegetables, fruits, raw nuts, raw seeds, whole grains and legumes—which can help detoxify estrogen. Eat essential fatty acids like flaxseed oil and hemp seed oil. Eat foods that are high in sulfur-rich amino acids—garlic, onions and beans.

Reduce or eliminate dairy products, eggs, red meat, sugar, white flour, refined foods, caffeine, chocolate, black and green teas and bad fat, all of which can increase estrogen. Avoid storing foods in, or eating foods from, plastic containers: plastic has been shown to increase estrogen in the body.

Vitamin C: *1 to 5 grams or more per day of buffered vitamin C with food. Some use more.*

And/or

SAMe: *400 to 1,500 mg per day in divided dosages. Start slowly and build up the dosage bi-weekly. Don't use with other SSRIs or herbs that increase serotonin without supervision.*

Detoxifying herbs: *Milk thistle, dandelion root, black radish, artichoke, burdock, yellow dock, wild yam, nettle and Oregon grape root all detoxify. Choose one or more from the list and take 40 drops of each three times per day on an empty stomach.*

Chastetree berry: *3 to 6 grams of the dried and ground berries three times a day; of the tincture, 30 drops three times per day. Chastetree berry is often standardized for 0.5 percent agnuside. If you are using a standardized tablet, take 175 to 225 mg daily; if a liquid extract, take ½ teaspoon (2 mL) a day.*

Topical use: *Poke root tincture and/or castor oil packs: five times per week.*

Acupuncture: *Regular acupuncture is excellent for cysts and fibroids.*

Multivitamin and mineral: *A good quality multivitamin and mineral: 1 per day with food.*

This may be all you need to bring your body back into balance. However, you may also want to consider some additional support:

Beta carotene: *50,000 IU a day with food.*

Selenium: *200 mcg with food.*

Vitamin E: *400 to 800 IU a day with food.*

Lipotropic factors: *1,000 mg of choline and inositol a day with food.*

Vaginal boluses: *5 times per week.*

Red clover: *Drink an infusion of 2 to 3 tsp (10 mL to 15 mL) per cup (250 mL) of water three times a day. If you prefer, you can take anywhere from 40 to 80 drops of the tincture three times a day, or 2 to 4 grams in pill form each day.*

Soy: *Enjoy freely in your diet.*

Fennel: *40 to 80 drops three times a day.*

Licorice: *If using the powder, take 1 to 2 grams three times a day; if using the fluid extract (1:1), take ½ to 1 tsp (4 mL) three times a day; if using the solid dry powdered extract (4:1), take 250 to 500 mg three times a day.*

Alfalfa: *500 to 1,000 mg per day in pill form.*

Motherwort: *40 drops three to four times a day on an empty stomach. In pill form, take 4½ grams a day on an empty stomach.*

Blue cohosh: *40 drops three to four times a day on an empty stomach.*

Black cohosh: *40 drops three to four times a day on an empty stomach.*

Red raspberry: *40 drops three to four times a day on an empty stomach. For the tea, infuse 1 to 2 tsp (5 mL to 10 mL) in 1 cup (250 mL) of water and drink freely one to three cups a day.*

Blue vervain: *30 drops of the tincture three times a day on an empty stomach, or infuse 1 tsp (4 mL) in a cup (250 mL) of water and drink three times a day on an empty stomach.*

Lady's mantle: *Make an infusion of 2 tsp (10 mL) of the herb per cup (250 mL) of water and drink three cups a day on an empty stomach.*

Please note: *If a cyst ruptures, you may need medical attention. Very large fibroids that press on organs may also require medical treatment.*

A typical herbal formula that combines help from all angles:

Try using detoxifying herbs like milk thistle, dandelion root, black radish, artichoke, burdock, yellow dock, wild yam and Oregon grape root or nettle; detoxifiers and anti-inflammatory herbs like turmeric; lymph drainers like red root, echinacea and cleavers; and growth shrinkers like chapparal, shiitake mushrooms, reishi mushrooms, and pau d'arco. Pick one or two herbs from each category, and use forty drops of each, in tincture or liquid extract form, 3 to 4 times a day on an empty stomach.

12

Help for Endometriosis

As many as one in thirty women suffers from endometriosis; yet we rarely hear about this disease. Perhaps the silence is because it often takes a long time to have the illness diagnosed and because diagnosis can be difficult and often involves surgery (called a laparoscopy). Laparoscopies are not always performed right away, as surgery should not be performed lightly. Doctors don't always diagnose endometriosis even when women describe symptoms of the illness. Although it is not generally believed that endometriosis causes infertility, many women with endometriosis also suffer from infertility. It seems that whatever is causing the one is also causing the other. It is important to get endometriosis correctly diagnosed for proper treatment and to prevent scarring which may be linked to infertility.

Symptoms

Common symptoms of endometriosis are: pelvic pain, painful periods, painful intercourse, painful bowel movements, intestinal discomfort, bleeding between periods, irregular menstrual flow and infertility.

Causes

Endometriosis occurs when small pockets of the uterus lining grow outside the uterus and in the pelvic area, the bowels, on the pelvic floor, in the bladder and in the ovaries. Endometrial tissue has shown up in noses and legs. These growths cause pain, irritation and scarring.

Some people believe a weakened immune system is behind the illness; others believe endometriosis is an autoimmune disease, or that it's caused by backed-up menstrual blood or an embryonic defect in cell differentiation, or that it's caused by candida. Candida expert Dr. Orion Truss explains that there is a very high association between endometriosis and candida, and says once the candida is treated, symptoms of endometriosis show dramatic decreases.

Damage caused by free radicals may be involved in some aspects of the disease. And, finally, an excessive estrogen-to-progesterone balance can lead to endometriosis. There is also a connection between pesticides and endometriosis. Many industrial chemicals mimic estrogen in the body.

Though we can't seem to agree about what causes endometriosis, many people think it's an estrogen-sensitive disease. Therefore, natural treatments aim to lower estrogen levels. Sound familiar? You can adjust your estrogen levels by looking at your diet and by using herbs and nutrients that balance hormones, reduce inflammation and support your liver.

Conventional Treatments

Conventional medicine generally finds and treats endometriosis with surgery. Some experts say the diagnostic surgery—laparoscopy—may cause endometriosis, since the instruments touching the inside of the abdomen may cause endometrial tissue to grow where it is not supposed to be. Some doctors have reported complete success using a treatment procedure called near-contact laparoscopy, which removes typical and atypical lesions.

Foods that Heal

A Vegetarian Diet

Diet is extremely important in treating endometriosis. Some women completely relieve their symptoms by following a vegetarian diet or a macrobiotic diet.

Eat Your Iodine and Other Healing Foods

Foods high in iodine are important in treating this disease; a deficiency of iodine can trigger the illness. Eat foods like kelp, dulse, hijki and non. It is also important to eat greens like swiss chard, turnip greens and watercress, which are all healing foods.

Eat Whole Foods

Try to eat whole grains—in your pasta, bread and rice. Whole grains are excellent sources of vitamins B and E, which are needed to balance hormones through their effects on the liver and ovaries. Whole grains are also full of minerals that prevent cramping; they're high in protein; and they contain lots of fiber, which removes excess estrogen and normalizes bowel movements. Also try legumes—soy (tofu, soy burgers, soy dogs), lentils, chickpeas (hummus) and kidney beans (yummy chili). Legumes are rich in minerals—including those that are lost through heavy bleeding—in B vitamins, in protein and in fiber. Vegetables, seeds and nuts are also excellent in treating endometriosis, as they can lower estrogen levels.

Eat Your Essential Fatty Acids

Essential fatty acids (EFAs) produce anti-inflammatory prostaglandins, and prostaglandin imbalances often accompany endometriosis. So take 1 to 2 tablespoons

(15 mL to 30 mL) of flaxseed oil, hemp oil, sunflower oil or walnut oil every day to reduce inflammation.

Things to Avoid

Meat and all dairy products make excess estrogen in the body, which can make you susceptible to endometriosis. Avoid chocolate, coffee, salt, sugar, fried foods and processed foods: all contribute to endometriosis. Avoid alcohol, which stresses your liver and has been associated with high estrogen levels.

Herbs and Supplements that Help

Antioxidants: Vitamin C, Bioflavonoids, Vitamins E and A

Antioxidants help to reduce free radical damage that may be involved in endometriosis. Vitamin C and bioflavonoids, both antioxidants, help reduce heavy bleeding and also help your body absorb iron, which you need because you lose iron when you bleed. Flavonoids have an extra benefit: they're estrogenic, but they're much weaker than the estrogens in your body, so they can lower estrogen when necessary by stealing a receptor site from your body's stronger estrogen. Vitamin A, or beta-carotene, and vitamin E help keep your hormones balanced and are helpful for bleeding. Beta-carotene also enhances immunity and protects against growths; vitamin E prevents the inflammation that accompanies endometriosis.

Dosages
- Vitamin C: 2,000 mg three times a day with food. Use the calcium ascorbate form: it's more absorbable.
- Bioflavonoids: 1,000 to 2,000 mg of bioflavonoids a day with food.
- Vitamin A: 10,000 IU of vitamin A, or beta-carotene, with food every day.
- Vitamin E: 400 to 1,000 IU of a mixed tocopherol form of vitamin E with food. Mixed tocopherols are superior to the more commonly used alpha-tocopherol. Make sure your vitamin E is natural.

B Vitamins

The liver needs a good supply of B vitamins to eliminate excess estrogen. Balanced estrogen levels are crucial for treating endometriosis

Dosage: 100 mg of a B-complex three times a day with food.

Iron

You need to take iron to replace the iron you lose during heavy bleeding.

Dosage: If a blood test determines that you need iron, take a non-constipating form of iron; for example, Floradix, or iron bound to succinate or fumarate, with food. Dosage is best worked out with a practitioner.

Calcium, Magnesium and Potassium

Calcium, magnesium and potassium can help prevent the painful cramping that comes with endometriosis. The calcium and magnesium are best taken in a well-absorbed form, for example, citrate or kreb's cycle. You can get good potassium from a kelp tablet.

Dosages

- Calcium: 1,500 mg every day of calcium in a well-absorbed form like citrate or kreb's cycle.
- Magnesium: 600 to 1,000 mg of magnesium in a well-absorbed form like citrate or kreb's cycle.
- Potassium: Potassium, as well as other minerals, including extra iodine, can be obtained by taking one to two kelp tablets one to three times a day. Dosage is best determined by a practitioner.

Hormone Balance

Natural Progesterone Cream

Natural progesterone cream can offset the estrogen dominance in your body and has no dangerous side effects. (Synthetic hormones can have dangerous side effects.)

Dosages: One half-teaspoon of the cream is usually applied morning and night to the soft parts of the body on a rotating basis, at different times of the cycle. The dosage is often individual. See a practitioner for this supplement.

Chastetree Berry

Chastetree berry balances estrogen and progesterone levels. Herbal expert Christopher Hobbes reports that German gynecologists are having remarkable success using chastetree berry to treat endometriosis

Dosage: Three to six grams of the dried and ground berries three times a day; of the tincture, 30 drops three times a day. Chastetree berry is often standardized for 0.5 percent agnuside. If you are using a standardized tablet, take 175 to 225 mg daily; if a liquid extract, take ½ teaspoon (2 mL) a day.

Liver Support

Liver support is one of the main focuses in the treatment of endometriosis. The liver not only excretes estrogen, it also breaks it down into a safer form that doesn't cause tissue growth. Try milk thistle, oregano, ginger root, boldo, articoke, wild yam, yellow dock or dandelion root.

Dosages: 30 to 40 drops of one or each three to four times per day.

Inflammation

Black Cohosh, Prickly Ash

Herbs like black cohosh and prickly ash stimulate circulation to the pelvic region; they also help clear out inflammation, adhesions and stagnation, so they can help in the treatment of endometriosis

Dosages: 40 drops of black cohosh and/or prickly ash half an hour before meals three to four times per day.

Castor Oil Packs

Castor oil packs are particularly useful for endometriosis. Castor oil packs are applied for three consecutive nights, for an hour, every week until the condition improves. See page 93 in Chapter 11.

Astringent Herbs

Shepherd's Purse, Yarrow, Nettle

Use any or all of these three herbs if bleeding is a particular problem. Their astringent properties will help dry up excess bleeding.

Dosages
- Shepherd's purse: 40 drops three times per day, or every half-hour if bleeding is severe, on an empty stomach.
- Nettle: 40 to 150 drops three to four times per day on an empty stomach. For pill or tea forms, take 2 to 5 grams three times per day on an empty stomach.
- Yarrow: 40 to 100 drops three times per day on an empty stomach. For the pill form take 4½ grams per day on an empty stomach. As a tea, take an infusion of 1 to 2 tsp (5 mL to 10 mL) three times per day on an empty stomach.

Strengthening the Body

Eleuthero, Nettle

Many women who suffer from endometriosis develop anemia. Eleuthero (formerly known as Siberian ginseng) is a strengthening and energizing herb. Nettle tea will also help you regain your strength because it supplies iron to replace lost iron stores.

Dosages

- Eleuthero: 5 to 15 grams per day on an empty stomach.
- Nettle: Infuse 2 to 5 grams for each cup of water; drink three cups a day on an empty stomach.

THE SUPER HERBAL COMBINATION: PUTTING IT TOGETHER

Drink as much of this incredible herbal tea as you like. It can effectively and safely treat endometriosis. Keep the herbs in the following ratios:

- 3 parts dandelion root
- 3 parts wild yam
- 2 parts burdock root
- 2 parts pau d'arco
- 1 part Oregon grape root
- 1 part chastetree berry
- ½ part dong quai

Use 4 to 6 tablespoons (60 mL to 90 mL) of the herb mixture for each quart (liter) of water, and decoct for twenty minutes. Drink three to four times a day. You will be amazed by the results: these herbs are an incredible combination for endometriosis because they balance your hormones, help your liver and digestive system, are antispasmodic, have anti-inflammatory properties and can help shrink growths!

Finally an End to Endometriosis

Women who've been suffering from endometriosis don't have to suffer any more. They can lead very normal, productive and healthy lives by rebalancing the hormones and correcting the underlying problems using natural herbs, diet and supplements.

The Protocol for Treating Endometriosis

Follow the dietary suggestions given in this chapter. Some women completely relieve their symptoms by following a vegetarian diet or a macrobiotic diet. Focus on foods that are rich in iodine and essential fatty acids, and eat whole foods; avoid alcohol, meat, dairy products, caffeine, excess sugar and salt, and deep-fried and processed foods. Avoid plastics and chemicals as much as possible.

Chastetree berry: *The usual dosage of chastetree berry is 3 to 6 grams of the dried and ground berries three times a day; of the tincture, 30 drops three times a day. Chastetree berry is often standardized for 0.5 percent agnuside. If you are using a standardized tablet, take 175 to 225 mg daily; if a liquid extract, take ½ teaspoon (2 mL) a day.*

And/or

Progesterone cream: *Dosage: One half teaspoon of the cream is usually applied morning and night to the soft parts of the body on a rotating basis, at different times of the cycle. The dosage is often individual. See a practitioner for this supplement.*

The Super Herbal Combination: *given in this chapter. Enjoy it three to four times per day on an empty stomach.*

Castor oil packs: *Use three to four times per week.*

High-potency multivitamin and mineral: *Take one a day with food.*

This may be all you need to bring your body back into balance. However, you may also want to consider some additional support:

B-vitamins: *100 mg three times a day, with food,*

Vitamin C: *2,000 mg of calcium ascorbate (a more absorbable vitamin C) three times a day with food.*

Bioflavonoids: *1,000 to 2,000 mg per day with food.*

Beta-carotene or vitamin A: *10,000 IU a day with food.*

Iron: *Use a non-constipating from of iron, for example, Floradix, or iron bound to succinate or fumarate, with food. Use if needed, as determined by a blood test.*

Vitamin E: *400 to 1,000 IU of natural mixed tocopherol vitamin E with food.*

Calcium: *1,500 mg a day with food, preferably a well-absorbed form, such as a citrate or kreb's cycle.*

Magnesium: *1,000 mg a day with food, preferably from a well-absorbed source such as a citrate or kreb's cycle.*

Kelp: *Dosage is best determined by a practitioner.*

Further Help

Excessive Bleeding

Shepherd's purse: *40 drops, three times per day, or every half-hour if bleeding is severe, on an empty stomach.*

Nettle: *40 to 150 drops three to four times per day on an empty stomach. For the pill or tea forms, take 2 to 5 grams three times per day on an empty stomach.*

Yarrow: *40 to 100 drops three times per day on an empty stomach. For the pill form, take 4½ grams per day on an empty stomach. As a tea, drink an infusion of 1 to 2 tsp (5 to 10 mL) three times per day on an empty stomach.*

Anemia and Low Energy

Eleuthero (formerly Siberian ginseng): *5 to 15 grams per day on an empty stomach. For energy.*

Nettle tea: *Drink an infusion of 1 to 2 tsp (5 mL to 10 mL) three times per day on an empty stomach. For anemia.*

Inflammation

Black cohosh and prickly ash: *40 drops of black cohosh and or prickly ash half an hour before meals 3 to 4 times per day, on an empty stomach. Reduces inflammation, adhesions and stagnation.*

For further help, see the above chapter.

13

Safe Help for Pregnancy

For centuries, women all over the world have used herbs safely to have healthy pregnancies. Herbs can help with pregnancy and many of the illnesses that just happen to occur when a woman is pregnant. Herbs can help bring the body, including the hormones, back into balance. (Note: Dosages are only given in this chapter where they are generic. It is best to consult a natural health practitioner for dosages and herbs best for you.)

Herb Supreme for Pregnancy: Red Raspberry Leaf

Red raspberry leaf has been called the "herb supreme for pregnancy." It is a wonderful tonic that helps prepare the uterus for birth: it relaxes and relieves cramps. It's so effective that many women report virtually pain-free labors thanks to red raspberry leaf tea!

Red raspberry leaf is rich in iron, calcium, potassium and vitamins B, C and E. Studies show it helps with morning sickness and postpartum depression, prevents bleeding at birth, prevents hemorrhaging, returns the uterus to normal quickly after birth and encourages breast milk. It is safe to take and without side effects.

Dosage: Make an infusion of 1 tsp (5 mL) of red raspberry leaf per cup (250 mL) of boiling water; cover for twenty minutes, then strain. Drink three cups a day on an empty stomach, half an hour before each meal. It is traditionally used during the last three months of pregnancy on a daily basis.

Relief from Morning Sickness

There are many safe and effective herbs that can be used for nausea during pregnancy. Herbalists Rosemary Gladstar, author of *Herbal Healing for Women*, and Amanda McQuade Crawford, author of *Herbal Remedies for Women*, suggest peppermint, slippery elm, chamomile flowers, lemon balm, small amounts of dandelion root and—the real herbal superstar for nausea—ginger.

Ginger

Ginger has a long history of relieving nausea, including morning sickness. This traditional use has now been confirmed in studies.[1] Even for the severe form of morning sickness called *hyperemesis gravidarum*, ginger is the herb to use. In one study of thirty women with this condition, 250 mg of ginger four times a day safely reduced the severity of nausea and the number of vomiting attacks in 70 percent of subjects.[2]

Dosage: Ginger can be taken as a tea, or as a pill in dosages of up to 250 mg, four times a day.

GINGER CONTROVERSY?

Recently, there have been claims that ginger can cause birth defects and abortions. These controversial results were made only after an isolated compound of ginger was used rather than ginger as a whole food. Two studies found that the isolated compound may cause birth defects. The studies ignored the fact that other parts of ginger contain equally powerful antimutagenic properties. A 1991 review of the scientific literature found no reports of miscarriage or birth defects associated with ginger.[3] A more recent review of all the studies on ginger also could not find evidence that ginger harmed the mother or the child.[4] In other words, using ginger as a whole herb is not dangerous. In fact, the FDA considers five grams of ginger to be safe as a food, and only one gram is necessary during even the most severe form of nausea. Leading natural health expert Michael Murray, ND, reports that for the nausea and vomiting of pregnancy, ginger is safer to use than the antiemetic drugs prescribed by doctors, which can cause fetal abnormalities!

Slippery Elm

Slippery elm is one of my favorite herbs for an upset stomach. It not only settles an upset stomach, it also provides excellent nutrition.

Dosage: Mix 1 tsp (5 mL) or more of slippery elm powder per one cup (250 mL) of hot water, and drink as needed on an empty stomach. Use as much as you need, there is no top dose.

Herbs for Preventing Miscarriage

There are many herbs that help prevent miscarriages but do not interfere with the natural process of miscarriage when the fetus is damaged or improperly secured.[5] Useful herbs include false unicorn root, red raspberry, chastetree berry and wild yam. My two favorite herbs for preventing miscarriage are black haw and cramp bark.

Black Haw

One of the best herbs for preventing miscarriage is black haw. It's been used for centuries, is still used in Europe, and it's powerful enough to counteract even the effect of abortion drugs.

Black haw contains several powerful uterine relaxants. It works by reducing the severity of contractions, and you can use it to relieve uterine cramping all through your pregnancy. It causes relaxation only when contractions are excessive; it doesn't interfere with the normal contractions of labor. It can also prevent abortions. Like aspirin, it contains salicins, which give it painkilling properties.

Cramp Bark

Cramp bark, a near relative of black haw, has many of the same components and is used in much the same way. This antispasmodic is especially helpful in preventing miscarriages resulting from stress or anxiety, and it can be safely used over time to treat threatened miscarriages. There are no side effects.

Herbs and Supplements for Preeclempsia

Preeclempsia is a serious condition that can occur in pregnant women, where blood pressure is elevated, fluid is retained, and there is loss of protein in the urine. It occurs in the third trimester.

Spirulina and Dandelion Leaf

Spirulina and dandelion leaf, diuretics rich in potassium, are great herbs for treating and preventing preeclempsia.

Hawthorn and Nettle

Nettle and hawthorn are also used to treat and prevent preeclempsia. Hawthorn, a diuretic and an antioxidant, helps lower blood pressure. Nettle is a diuretic that supports the kidney and is rich in calcium, magnesium and vitamin C—three crucial nutrients for preventing preeclempsia. The two herbs also support the liver and kidneys, which can help with preeclempsia.

Vitamins and Minerals

Calcium, magnesium, beta-carotene, vitamin E and vitamin C play a huge role in treating preeclampsia. Women with preeclempsia are often calcium deficient.[6] When women are at high risk for preeclempsia, taking calcium supplements is very effective at reducing that risk.[7]

Magnesium deficiency can also cause preeclempsia. If you are at high risk, supplementing with magnesium can lower that risk. [8]

Women with preeclempsia are also low in antioxidants.[9] In women at high risk for preeclempsia, double-blind research has found that taking 1 g of vitamin C and 400 IU of vitamin E reduces the risk by an incredible 76 percent.[10]

Herbal Superstars for Bringing On Birth

Blue Cohosh and Black Cohosh

These are good and safe herbs to take when it is time for birth, either because labor has begun or a health professional has determined that it is time. (They should not be used earlier in the pregnancy since they could cause a miscarriage.)

In the last week of pregnancy, black cohosh can help your body prepare for labor or can bring on an overdue labor. It has been used this way by aboriginal healers for countless years. It stimulates contractions while relaxing tension in the uterine muscles, easing the pain of labor. Blue cohosh also helps bring on contractions when labor is prolonged or so overdue it has become risky.

Motherwort

Motherwort prepares the uterus for labor, brings on contractions and eases the birth.

Herbs to Relax Excess Cramping During Birth

Cramp Bark

Simply put, cramp bark works by safely relaxing uterine muscles and is a wonderful herb to take before and during labor to ease cramping without interfering with the birth process.

Black Haw

This uterine tonic safely quiets uterine muscles and eases the tension that comes with contractions.

Valerian and Chamomile

Valerian and chamomile flowers are great relaxant herbs that ease excessive spasming and the cramps of labor.

Herbs to Stop Bleeding

If there is bleeding after delivery, try packing the affected area with yarrow or shepherd's purse, or drink an infusion of these two herbs.

Herbs to Heal Tears and Damaged Tissue

For tears, try packing comfrey root into the area. Warning: comfrey should be used only externally. Midwives and herbalists can prepare these herbs specifically for you.

Treating Colds and Flues While Pregnant

There are many safe and effective treatments for colds and flues during pregnancy.

Immune Boosters

When you're pregnant vitamin C, echinacea, garlic and elderberry are amazing supplements to take for colds and the flu. Vitamin C builds immunity; it can prevent and treat colds and the flu. Echinacea is the great immune-building herb and also prevents and treats the flu and colds. Garlic fights viruses, and can be used for prevention and treatment. Elderberry stops viruses from replicating, which means it can stop a cold or flu dead in its tracks.

Diaphoretics

Lemon balm is great for fighting viruses, as are chamomile, catnip, linden, ginger and peppermint. They are diaphoretics that encourage your body's immune system and help it fight off viruses.

Further Help for Colds and Flues

Other remedies for colds and flues include sage and slippery elm. Sage is great as a gargle for a sore throat. Slippery elm is great for sore throats and upset stomachs. Try drinking lemon and honey tea or gargling with warm salt water for colds. Or place a few drops of eucalyptus essential oil in hot water and inhale the steam.

Constipation

Countless pregnant women suffer from constipation. There are many nutrients that can help relieve constipation.

Fiber

Start with ground flaxseeds and other foods rich in fiber, and drink lots of water. Eat raw greens, raw seeds, nuts, fruit, legumes and whole grains.

Prunes

The fruit and the juice are both great remedies. Eat or drink as needed, as determined by a practitioner.

Probiotics

Acidophilus can also help correct the problem.

Herbal Help

Yellow dock and dandelion are very good remedies for constipation. I especially like yellow dock—it's a good, safe solution, and can also be used for anemia.

Sleeping

Don't suffer through sleepless nights—there are lots of wonderful natural and safe ways to have a good night's rest when you're pregnant.

Calcium and Magnesium

For insomnia and anxiety, try calcium and magnesium. These minerals are great for relaxing, and they can reduce anxiety and stress.

Herbal Help

Valerian, skullcap, passionflower, lavender, catnip, lemon balm, linden and St. John's wort are always great herbal choices for relaxing and sleeping. St. John's wort is especially good if you also suffer from depression, and passionflower and valerian are especially good if your insomnia comes with anxiety.

Scented Sleep

Try a hops and/or lavender pillow: Fill a pillow with a little lavender and/or hops and sleep on it or near it.

With a little help from nature, you can prevent and treat problems and have a healthy, happy pregnancy. No sample protocol is given here, as it is best to work with a natural healer when you are pregnant, in order to tailor a unique approach to you.

14

How to Have a Healthy, Happy Menopause

E very woman will at some point in her life go through menopause. The question is how to do it with ease and comfort. How you have lived your life up to the time of menopause can sometimes determine how comfortable or uncomfortable menopause will be, and how well you've balanced your hormones throughout your life can make all the difference when you reach menopause. But don't worry, the natural approach can help every woman go through menopause safely and easily. With a few easy-to-make changes, you can enjoy a healthy, happy menopause.

And remember, menopause is not a disease: it is a natural process that every woman will go through, and on the other side there is freedom and creativity.

Symptoms

Much of the media coverage of menopause treats it as if it is a disease. Menopause is not a disease, but a natural progression in a woman's life. Yet women who live in a western culture, with all its bad habits, often experience uncomfortable and disturbing changes when they go through menopause: hot flashes, night sweats, palpitations and insomnia, vaginal dryness and thinning, depression and other problems.

But woman do not need to suffer, nor do they need to go on dangerous chemical hormones to get relief. Natural health offers safe and effective relief. Diet and lifestyle are crucial to a healthy, symptom-free menopause. And, for women who need a little extra help, there are a number of super herbs that work wonders.

Foods that Heal

Women who have a diet that is rich in whole foods, like fresh vegetables, whole grains, legumes, raw seeds, nuts and fruits, have an easier time in menopause. A whole-food diet provides better nutrition and creates less toxic buildup.

Try eating a vegetarian diet that is high in fiber, antioxidants and essential fatty acids, for example, flaxseed oil, and low in unhealthy hydrogenated fats. Antioxidants, like vitamins E and C, fiber and essential fatty acids can help you have a healthier, happier menopause.

Try to include more phtyoestrogenic foods; for example, soy, fennel, celery, parsley, flaxseeds and other raw seeds and nuts. These foods reduce the symptoms of menopause. It's easy too: have a soy burger; eat tabbouleh (a Middle Eastern parsley salad—and one of my favorites); make a Thai stir fry loaded with tofu; use flaxseeds in soy smoothies, muffins and on hot cereals.

To reduce the hot flashes that can come with menopause, cut down on or avoid alcohol, caffeine and sugar.

These simple changes can make you feel better surprisingly quickly. In fact, you can feel even better than you did before you reached menopause, because eating these foods puts less strain on your system, reduces toxins and supplies crucial nutrients.

Excercise, Stress Reduction and Cleansing

Exercising throughout your life can greatly ease menopausal symptoms, and it helps build your bones. Periodic internal cleansing of the body throughout life can also aid menopause. And don't forget to do something to relieve stress: walk, run, do yoga, meditate, take a break. Do whatever works for you.

Herbs that Help

Isoflavones

Isoflavones, nutrients found in soy, are weakly estrogenic, meaning they have an incredible ability: they gently raise your estrogen if your levels are low (as in menopause), but, if your estrogen levels are too high (as in breast cancer), isoflavones can lower estrogen levels by stealing receptor sites from your own more powerful estrogen. Studies have shown soy isoflavones help not only with hot flashes, but also with vaginal dryness and thinning, breast cancer, osteoporosis and the psychological symptoms of menopause.

Soy

Drink one glass or more of soy milk a day, and try edamame (steamed soybeans) as a snack—it's delicious!

Red Clover

A recent study found that red clover, another source of isoflavones, may have cardiovascular benefits for menopausal women.[1]

> **Dosage:** Take 40 to 80 drops of red clover as a tincture three times per day on an empty stomach. As a pill, take 2 to 4 grams per day. If the pill is standardized for 40 mg isoflavones, take 1 to 2 grams per day.

Herbal Superstar: Black Cohosh

This native North American plant is a herbal superstar for menopausal women.

In Germany, black cohosh is used more than any other herb for menopause, and for good reason. Black cohosh is so remarkable that it consistently outperforms estrogen therapy in the treatment of menopause.[2] And, unlike the hormones, it works safely and without side effects.

It is wonderfully effective as a treatment for hot flashes, sweating and heart palpitations. It can help treat vaginal thinning and dryness[3]—problems that estrogen has little effect on. Studies have also shown that black cohosh is extremely effective—better than hormones or Valium—in treating the nervousness, irritability, depression, anxiety and sleep disturbances that can accompany menopause.[4] The herb may also be able to help with the osteoporosis associated with menopause.[5]

Black cohosh, like isoflavones, has an advantage over estrogen therapy: it doesn't stimulate breast tumors. Quite the opposite, in fact: it markedly inhibits breast tumors[6], unlike chemical estrogens, which are believed to cause breast cancer.

Dosage: Use an extract standardized for 1 mg of the triterpine 27-deoxyacteine in each tablet; take 2 tablets, or 40 drops if it's a liquid, twice a day. If the herb is not standardized, take ½ to 1 gram three to four times a day on an empty stomach.

The Queen of Herbs for Women: Chastetree Berry

The queen of female tonics, this herb is the great hormone balancer: it balances the ratio of estrogen to progesterone and helps treat some of the underlying causes of many of the uncomfortable symptoms of menopause. It slightly favors progesterone over estrogen. Often, progesterone's role in relieving menopause is overlooked, yet most menopausal women have low progesterone. This incredible herb also helps with vaginal dryness, hot flashes, dizziness and the depression that often accompanies menopause.

Dosage: The usual dosage of chastetree berry is 3 to 6 grams of the dried and ground berries three times a day; of the tincture, 30 drops three times a day. Chastetree berry is often standardized for 0.5 percent agnuside. If you are using a standardized tablet, take 175 to 225 mg daily; if a liquid extract, take ½ tsp (2mL) a day.

Dong Quai

This herb has a long history in China as a female remedy. Dong quai is a cardiovascular and hormonal tonic; it's also a nervine (a herb used for toning nerves), which makes it a useful herb in any menopause formula. It's sometimes called "the female ginseng." Dong quai normalizes hormones by acting on the blood vessels, the liver and the endocrine system. It is a strengthening and nourishing herb that is good for easing into menopause and for difficulties that arise during menopause like hot flashes.

> **Dosage:** 1 to 5 grams taken as tea three times per day on an empty stomach. In pill form, take 1 to 4 grams three times per day on an empty stomach. As a tincture, take ½ tsp to 1 tsp (2 to 4 mL), and as an extract take ¼ tsp (1 mL) three times per day, both on an empty stomach.

Wild Yam

Wild yam normalizes hormone production and regulates the balance of estrogen and progesterone, making it a useful herb for menopause. Since it helps the liver, wild yam is especially useful when not only the reproductive system, but also the liver is behind the hormone imbalance. Wild yam contains steroidal precursors that your body may use in a similar manner to its own hormones.

> **Dosage:** One gram of dried powdered root three times per day. As a tincture, take ½ tsp to 1 tsp (2 mL to 4 mL) three times per day on an empty stomach.

Licorice

The use of licorice dates back many centuries, and it has been used in both the East and the West. Licorice is believed to possess estrogen-like properties, which makes it a wonderful herb for treating menopause. It also is believed to raise progesterone levels: another important benefit for women in menopause. It is a great herb for getting rid of hot flashes and depression.

> **Dosage:** 1 to 2 grams of the root as tea, 2 to 3 cups a day. If you prefer the extract, take ½ tsp to 1 tsp (2 mL to 4 mL) three times a day. As a pill (4:1 solid extract) take 250 to 500 mg three times a day on an empty stomach.

Sage

For women who suffer from hot flashes, sage can offer a special benefit. Because it is an astringent herb, it can dry up hot flashes, especially night sweats. I have seen this simple tea do wonders time and time again.

> **Dosage:** 3 cups of the tea per day (made as a herbal infusion) on an empty stomach.

Liver Herbs: Dandelion Root and Milk Thistle

The liver is an important organ for the production, regulation and detoxification of hormones. Therefore, herbs that work on the liver, like dandelion, yellow dock, boldo and milk thistle, are great herbs for menopause. Women who have had a poor diet or consumed excess alcohol and caffeine should especially take liver herbs prior to and during menopause.

Dosage: 40 drops, or more, of one or more of any of the above herbs in tinctures three to four times per day on an empty stomach.

Vitamins and Minerals

Vitamin E

Take vitamin E to fight hot flashes. It can be taken internally or used topically to fight vaginal dryness. Several studies show that vitamin E is effective in relieving hot flashes and menopausal vaginal complaints. [7]

Dosages: Up to 800 IU to 1,200 IU of natural, mixed vitamin E a day with food.

Vitamin C

Vitamin C, mixed with bioflavonoids, offers help for hot flashes. In one study, 87 percent of women who took vitamin C mixed with bioflavonoids experienced improvement in their hot flashes. [8]

Dosage: 1 to 3 grams of vitamin C per day mixed with bioflavonoids, with food.

Bone-Building Nutrients

All women should take bone-building nutrients: calcium, magnesium, zinc and manganese. These nutrients are even more crucial at menopause, as hormone levels begin to drop. See Chapter 15 for more information on bone health.

Dosage: 1,500 mg of calcium, 600 mg of magnesium, 25 mg of zinc and 1,000 IU (or more) of vitamin D, mixed with other bone-building nutrients, for example, manganese, a B-complex and vitamin C.

Multivitamin

Supplement your diet with a good-quality multivitamin and mineral complex. Extra nutrients can be a great aid during menopause—and, really, all through your life.

Finally, an End to Menopausal Difficulties

Menopause does not have to be spent in pain and discomfort. With a few changes, you'll be surprised at how good you feel. Many women find menopause a time of great liberation and growth. So spend some time on yourself, get some exercise and maybe do a little meditation or yoga. Tune in to your body and supply it with what it needs to make the transition so that this important time of your life is a happy, healthy and productive one.

Sample Protocol for Menopause

Eat whole foods and avoid empty, processed foods. Try eating a vegetarian diet that is high in fiber, antioxidants and essential fatty acids (for example, flaxseed oil) and low in unhealthy hydrogenated fats.

Focus on eating phtyoestrogenic foods, like soy foods, flaxseeds, celery, fennel and parsley. Get as much exercise as you can. To reduce the hot flashes that can come with menopause, cut down on or avoid alcohol, caffeine and sugar.

Black cohosh: *Get an extract standardized for 1 mg of the triterpine 27-deoxyacteine in each tablet, and take 2 tablets, or 40 drops if it's a liquid, twice a day. If the herb is not standardized, take half a gram to a gram three to four times per day on an empty stomach.*

High-potency multivitamin and mineral: *Take daily with food.*

Bone-building supplement: *Take 1,500 mg of calcium, 600 mg of magnesium, 25 mg of zinc, 1,000 IU or more of vitamin D, and add other bone-building nutrients, for example, manganese, a B-complex and vitamin C.*

Sage: *For help with hot flashes, drink an infusion of sage, three times per day on an empty stomach.*

If after one month, symptoms such as hot flashes and vaginal dryness are still present, try the following:

Vitamin E: *Use internally or topically to help fight vaginal dryness. Take up to 800 IU to 1,200 IU of natural, mixed vitamin E a day with food.*

Vitamin C with bioflavanoids: *To ease hot flashes, take 1 to 3 grams per day with food.*

If more help is needed after two to three months, try any one or more of the following:

Chastetree berry: *The usual dosage of chastetree berry is 3 to 6 grams of the dried and ground berries three times a day; of the tincture, 30 drops three times a day. Chastetree berry is often standardized for 0.5 percent agnuside. If you are using a standardized tablet, take 175 to 225 mg daily; if a liquid extract, take ½ tsp (2 mL) per day.*

Dong quai: *1 to 5 grams as a tea, three times per day on an empty stomach, or 1 to 4 grams in pill form three times per day on an empty stomach. As a tincture, take ½ tsp to 1 tsp (2 mL to 4 mL) three times per day; as an extract, take ¼ tsp (1 mL) three times per day.*

continued

Wild yam: *1 gram of dried powdered root three times per day on an empty stomach. As a tincture, take ½ tsp to 1 tsp (2 mL to 4 mL) three times per day on an empty stomach.*

Licorice: *On an empty stomach, take licorice in any of the following ways: of the dried, powdered root take 1 to 2 grams three times per day. As a tea, drink 2 to 3 cups per day. Of the extract, take ½ tsp to 1 tsp (2 mL to 4 mL) three times per day. As a pill (4:1 solid extract) take 250 to 500 mg three times per day.*

Red clover: *40 to 80 drops of the tincture three times per day on an empty stomach. As a pill, take 2 to 4 grams per day. If the pill is standardized for 40 mg isoflavones, take 1 to 2 grams per day.*

For those who need liver help *(anyone who is full of toxins or regularly consumes caffeine, alcohol or other empty foods):*

Try dandelion root and milk thistle. Take 40 to 80 drops of one or more of the tinctures three to four times per day on an empty stomach.

For the psychological symptoms of menopause:

Try one or more of black cohosh, chastetree berry, licorice and red clover. See pages 117 to 119 for dosages.

For palpitations:

Take black cohosh. See page 117 for dosage.

For vaginal dryness:

Try one or more of these supplements: red clover (see page 117), vitamin E (see page 120), black cohosh (see page 117), chastetree berry (see page 118).

For hot flashes:

Try one or more of these supplements: black cohosh (see page 117), chastetree berry (see page 118), red clover (see page 117), dong quai (see page 118), licorice (see page 119), sage (see page 119), vitamin C with flavonoids (see page 120), vitamin E (see page 120).

15

Prevention and Treatment of Osteoporosis

W e all know it's primarily women who have to worry about their bones. But did you know that osteoporosis and even osteopenia—its precursor—can start long before menopause? You set up your bone health by how well you eat, exercise and keep in balance when you're young. But it's never too late to start working on your bones, and natural health can go a long way toward building and maintaining your bones.

Bone health depends on a balanced body. It's linked to a healthy cycle and to healthy eating and exercise. High estrogen levels alone will not give you strong bones. Your hormones need to be balanced to make strong bones. The key is that estrogen and progesterone in balance help to make strong bones.

Geography and Bones

In some countries of the world, very few people develop osteoporosis. And we don't need to get it here, either, if we make some healthy changes. Yet in North America, osteoporosis continues to be the single most common bone disease, and 40 percent of all white women develop it in their lifetime. In North America, estrogen and milk are continually pushed as ways to prevent bone problems, yet clearly this approach is not working. Why? Let's take a look at what to do and what not to do for strong and healthy bones.

The Estrogen Myth

We are still being told that dropping estrogen levels at menopause are the cause of osteoporosis. But, in 1985, studies at the Mayo Clinic found that half of all vertebral bone loss takes place before menopause. Dr. Susan Brown, Ph.D., points out that if falling estrogen levels caused osteoporosis, all women would develop it, and they don't.

In several cultures, postmenopausal women have lower estrogen levels *and* less osteoporosis than women in the West. Vegetarian women have lower estrogen levels than meat eaters but *higher* bone density. Recent research found that estrogen levels in women with and without osteoporosis are the same.

Even more interesting, not one study using estrogen treatment alone has shown any lasting increase in bone mass. The reason is simple: although estrogen slows bone loss for the few years that it accelerates during menopause, the effect wears off a few years later, and estrogen cannot rebuild new bone. Women's estrogen levels *should* drop at menopause, since estrogen is no longer needed for reproduction, and artificially high levels increase the risk of breast cancer.

New studies link estrogen pills to heart disease (even in women with no history of previous heart disease) and cancer. It seems even more important that women not supplement estrogen.

Calcium Balance

Obviously, calcium is important to bone health. But bone health isn't about calcium intake—it's about calcium balance. In other words, it isn't how much calcium you take, it's also how much you're losing that matters.

In North America, most women get plenty of calcium, but they also take in many things that leach calcium from their bodies. How much calcium you need depends on how much calcium you lose. Studies show that Japanese women need only 550 mg of calcium a day, while North American women need 1,241 mg a day to offset the calcium they lose because of their diets. In many cultures where osteoporosis is virtually unheard of, people take in only 175 to 540 mg of calcium a day. The difference is that they don't take in much of the substances that leach calcium as North American women do.

What causes calcium loss? Excessive animal protein, sugar, phosphorus, caffeine, salt, tobacco, alcohol, cortisone and antibiotics.

Calcium Leachers

Eat as close to a vegetarian diet as you can for healthy, strong bones. Research shows that eliminating animal protein can reduce calcium loss by 50 percent, and that vegetarians have superior bone density. Part of the reason is that when the body breaks down protein, it produces acid, which must be buffered before it can be excreted. The body uses calcium to buffer it. That calcium is drawn from the bones. The more protein you eat, the more calcium you need.

Perhaps this is one reason a twelve-year study done at Harvard Medical School found that women who drank two or more glasses of milk a day had a 45 percent *higher* risk of hip fractures than women who drank less milk.[1] Milk is high in animal protein and contains phosphorus, which also leaches calcium.

Phosphorus is also found in meat and soft drinks. Of course soft drinks are also high in sugar and caffeine. Sugar reduces calcium absorption and increases the excretion of calcium and other key bone nutrients. The risk of hip fracture increases with caffeine consumption. Not surprisingly, drinking soft drinks has been linked to increased bone fractures.

Eating for Your Bones

For strong and healthy bones, try to eat whole foods that are high in bone-building nutrients: whole grains; legumes; raw seeds, such as sesame seeds, or tahini (a calcium-rich paste made from sesame seeds that is loaded in calcium); nuts; deep leafy greens, for example, kale, chard and bok choy; sea vegetables; and other vegetables and fruit.

Bone-Building Nutrients

Calcium

Every woman has heard that she should take calcium for her bones. The question is: how much and in what form? While the amount may very depending on the person's diet, in general, it is a good idea to take a well-absorbed calcium, for example, calcium citrate or a calcium bound to kreb's cycle intermediates every day. Take calcium with dinner, as it is better absorbed later in the day.

Dosage: 1,200 to 1,500 mg of calcium citrate or calcium bound to kreb's cycle intermediates.

Calcium's Partner: Magnesium

Calcium does not work alone: in fact, too much isolated calcium may cause deficiencies of magnesium, and low magnesium levels are associated with osteoporosis. Studies show that taking magnesium increases bone density. Magnesium helps you absorb calcium. It also helps you absorb vitamin C, and it helps you convert vitamin D into its active form: crucial nutrients for bone health. Magnesium also stimulates hormones that preserve bone, and it regulates hormones that break bone down.

Dosage: 300 mg of magnesium twice per day with food.

Vitamin D

Vitamin D has been underestimated for years. Very simply put, taking vitamin D builds your bones, and people who are low in it have poor bones. Calcium needs vitamin D to be absorbed and deposited in the bone. Vitamin D alone can increase your bone density. Taking calcium with vitamin D not only stops bone loss, it increases bone density.

Dosage: 1,000 to 1,500 IU a day with food. Also, go outside in the early or late sunlight hours, and exercise every day. Sunlight not only prevents bone loss, but it protects against the most common forms of cancer: breast, colon and prostate cancers. To lessen the risk of potential sun-exposure problems, such as skin cancer, limit your sun exposure to the early and later parts of the day, when the sun is not at its strongest.

Vitamin C

Vitamin C is essential for the synthesis and repair of bone. It also helps with calcium absorption and the effects of vitamin D and stimulates cells that build bone. Vitamin C helps calcium to be absorbed and deposited in bone tissue.

Dosage: Take at least 1,000 mg of a buffered vitamin C a day with food.

Vitamin K

Vitamin K helps produce osteocalcin, which helps attract calcium to bone tissue. Without vitamin K, bones would be as soft as chalk. Since vitamin K supplementation is not always available, the best way to get it is to eat plenty of leafy green vegetables and to drink green tea.

Friendly Flora

Antibiotics wipe out the friendly flora that produce vitamin K, so you may want to try taking probiotics to replenish the friendly flora, to help make vitamin K and to help with the absorption of bone-building nutrients.

Dosage: 2 to 20 billion live cells of acidophilus and bifidus a day on an empty stomach. The higher dosages are usually used for only short periods of time.

Boron

Boron is crucial for bone health. Studies show that just 3 mg a day of boron can prevent calcium and magnesium loss in postmenopausal women. But it is not always available everywhere. So, once again, the best way to get boron is through your diet. Eat lots of leafy greens, apples, cherries, almonds, hazelnuts, beans and pears. Or get your boron from nettle, one of the best bone-building herbs there is.

The Bs

Other important nutrients for the bones are B6, B12 and folic acid, the trio that prevents homocysteine. Homocysteine interferes with collagen cross-linking, which causes defective bones.

Dosage: Take a B-complex, 50 mg, three times per day with food.

Other Key Nutrients

Deficiencies of manganese can increase the breakdown of bone and decrease bone mineralization. Zinc is also important to bone health: it helps with calcium absorption and vitamin D activity.

Dosage: Take a bone-building formula that includes manganese and zinc daily.

Digestive Enzymes

If you're taking sufficient nutrients and yet still having bone trouble, look to your digestive system. Low digestive enzymes prevent the absorption and utilization of nutrients that build bone. Taking digestive enzymes can help, as can herbs like licorice, fennel and caraway. All improve poor digestive function and absorption.

Dosage: Take 1 to 2 wide-spectrum plant-digestive enzymes with each meal.

Also, take these digestion-supporting herbs on an empty stomach, away from bone building nutrients:

- Licorice: 1 to 2 grams as a decoction, two to three cups a day.
- Fennel: Drink three cups a day as a decoction.
- Caraway: Drink three cups a day as a decoction.

Herbal Teas for Bones

What could be easier than adding a great-tasting tea to your day? The following herbs are excellent promoters of bone health:

- Nettle: rich in silica, calcium, magnesium, vitamin D, vitamin K and boron
- Chamomile: rich in calcium
- Alfalfa: rich in minerals, vitamin D and vitamin K
- Dandelion: rich in silica, minerals, vitamin D and vitamn K, boron, calcium and B vitamins.

Dosage: Buy the herbs in the loose herbs section of health foods stores and prepare as infusions. These teas are highly absorbable and taste quite pleasant. Consume three to four cups a day for strong bones.

Chastetree Berry

If progesterone is low, especially in young women—another cause for poor bone health—take chastetree berry and/or progesterone cream to bring the hormones into balance and to help build bones. Low progesterone levels are linked to poor bone health. Progesterone helps calcium stay in the bones. Again, it is an issue of hormone balance. Low progesterone levels can be detected by blood tests.

Dosage: The usual dosage of chastetree berry is 3 to 6 grams of the dried and ground berries three times a day; of the tincture, 30 drops three times a day. Chastetree berry is often standardized for 0.5 percent agnuside. If you are using a standardized tablet, take 175 to 225 mg daily; if a liquid extract, take ½ tsp (2 mL) a day.

Finally, Hormone-Free Relief for Osteoporosis

Follow the sample protocol and explore the other herbs listed in this chapter to create the program that's right for you. Don't forget to exercise: exercise helps to maintain strong and healthy bones, and if you do it in the sunlight, you get vitamin D to help build your bones.

The Protocol for Bone Health

Follow the dietary suggestions given here and in Chapter 5. Eat whole foods, especially dark leafy greens, sea vegetables, tahini, seeds, nuts, whole grains, legumes, vegetables and fruit. Eat as close to a vegetarian diet as you can for healthy, strong bones. Drink green tea, rich in boron. Avoid excessive animal protein, sugar, phosphorus caffeine, salt, tobacco, alcohol, cortisone and antibiotics.

Calcium: *1,200 to 1,500 mg of calcium citrate or krebs cycle intermediates with dinner.*

Magnesium: *600 mg of magnesium, with food, at lunch and dinner.*

Vitamin D: *1,000 to 1,500 IU or more per day with food.*

Vitamin C: *1,000 mg of a buffered vitamin C with dinner.*

B-complex: *50 mg three times per day, with each meal.*

Bone-building combination: *Take a vitamin and mineral combination that has all the key nutrients, including zinc, boron, vitamin K and manganese: complete bone care in a bottle.*

This may be all you need to bring your body back into balance. However, you may also want to consider some additional support. Try one or more of:

Chastetree berry: *Balanced hormones are essential for bone health, so consider chastetree berry. The usual dosage of chastetree berry is 3 to 6 grams of the dried and ground berries three times a day; of the tincture, 30 drops three times a day. Chastetree berry is often standardized for 0.5% agnuside. If you are using a standardized tablet, take 175 to 225 mg daily; if a liquid extract, take ½ tsp (2 mL) a day. For hormone balance.*

Bone teas (nettle, alfalfa, chamomile and dandelion): *Make infusions and consume three to four cups per day of one or a combination of the herbs.*

Digestive enzymes: *1 to 2 wide-spectrum plant-based enzymes with each meal.*

continued

CHAPTER FIFTEEN

Probiotics: *2 to 20 billion live cells a day on an empty stomach. The higher dosages are usually used for short periods only.*

For further help see the above chapter.

16

Healthy Weight Loss

E ating for hormonal balance not only gets rid of PMS and other women's health concerns, it also helps you to reach and maintain your optimal weight in a healthy way. It allows you to keep to your healthy weight and promotes good health for life. So you can cure your PMS, bring your hormones into balance and lose weight easily while you are doing it. Not bad!

As described in the previous chapters, focusing on eating whole foods and avoiding empty foods will help prevent all of the major chronic diseases down the road. A basic rule: eat lots of healthy fiber, and you will lose excess weight. You'll find fiber in vegetables, sea vegetables, fruits, whole grains, legumes, raw seeds and raw nuts. Focus on vegetables: start every meal with a large salad or vegetable juice. Use olive oil to cook with and use essential fatty acids, such as flaxseed oil, in your salads. EFAs help you lose weight. And don't skip meals: skipping meals can cause weight gain. Drink plenty of water every day, eight glasses minimum, to help with weight loss.

Simple Tips for Weight Loss

1. Drink eight glasses of water a day.
2. Eat plenty of fiber every day.
3. Eat vegetables (salad/juice) at the beginning of meals to load you up with healthy, non-fattening nutrients and to fill you up faster.
4. Eat vegetables and fruits for snacks.
5. After meals, swish your mouth with water or brush your teeth right away. This signals to your brain that the meal is over.
6. Use apple cider vinegar in salad dressings.
7. Don't skip meals: missing a meal will slow your metabolism down, which will make you overeat at the next meal.
8. Overeating and eating sweets often masks a desire for affection or love. So get a hug instead, or give one. Kiss your cat or dog. Better yet, take your dog for a walk.
9. Don't eat in front of the TV: it causes overeating.
10. Drink water when you first begin to feel hungry: thirst signals can be confused with hunger signals. This confusion can lead to overeating.
11. Don't eat when you are bored. Ask yourself, Am I really hungry?
12. Put small portions on your plate. You can take more if needed, but studies show that if you put larger amounts of food on your plate you will overeat.

13. Eat with someone: you are less likely to overeat.

14. Keep healthy snacks ready to go: washed, cut up and in the fridge. Try celery sticks, cucumber, berries, radishes, grapefruit, pineapple, mango and peppers.

15. Walk for an hour every day. Make this part of your lifestyle. It will keep the weight off, the stress down, and keep you feeling energized and stimulated—and less in need of a binge. Find a friend to walk with: it helps. For me, the walk is often the best part of my day.

Supplements that Help

There are some great natural supplements you can take that are designed to help curb appetite, burn fat and increase metabolism, lean muscle and energy. Let's take a look at some of these weight-loss nutrients.

Crucial Chromium

The health benefits of this valuable trace mineral were discovered in 1957, when chromium was found to be essential to proper blood sugar control. Chromium is a key factor in glucose tolerance—in balancing your sugar levels. It works closely with insulin in transporting glucose into cells for metabolism. Without chromium, insulin action is blocked, and blood sugar levels become elevated. Studies show that supplementing the diet with chromium decreases fasting glucose levels; improves tolerance to glucose; lowers insulin levels; and increases HDL, or good cholesterol, while reducing total cholesterol and triglyceride levels. Chromium is necessary in the metabolism of carbohydrates, proteins and fats.

Studies have shown that chromium can lower body weight while it increases lean body mass and muscle, probably by increasing your body's sensitivity to insulin.[1] According to Michael Murray, ND, "Improving insulin sensitivity is an important goal in a weight loss program. Loss of insulin sensitivity is the hallmark feature of obesity. Chromium is a trace mineral necessary for the proper action of insulin on blood sugar control."[2]

One study revealed that people taking chromium lost an average of seven times more body fat than those taking a placebo.[3] Most North Americans are deficient in chromium, so supplementation with chromium is very important.

Dosage: The dosage varies from person to person, but the usual range is between 200 mcg and 600 mcg, with food. Start slowly and increase as needed, depending on your health history. I often use about 400 mcg to 600 mcg in my practice, and I would recommend working with a natural health-care practitioner so you get the right amount for you. Diabetics need to be monitored.

Garcinia Cambogia (Hydroxycitric acid)

Hydroxycitric acid (HCA) comes from the rind of the Malabar Tamarind (*Garcinia cambogia*), a fruit native to South India. It has a great effect on how your body regulates its metabolism of fat. HCA inhibits a liver enzyme, which prevents glucose from synthesizing fatty acids. Also HCA controls your appetite and your cravings for sweets.

HCA is a lipogenic inhibitor: it inhibits the formation and buildup of fats. It also has other ways of promoting weight loss. HCA has been shown in studies to significantly reduce food intake: in other words, it suppresses appetite. It also inhibits the enzyme activity of ATP-citrate lyase, which is responsible for converting carbohydrates and proteins into fat. If you consume more calories than you burn, the excess calories are stored in your liver and muscles in the form of glycogen. When glycogen stores are filled, the excess calories are converted to fat, and your brain sends out signals indicating hunger. HCA enhances the ability of your liver and muscles to store glycogen, which helps to reduce fat production. HCA also prevents the brain from sending out signals that indicate hunger, so you don't feel the need to eat. So three things are accomplished: more calories are burned as energy, fewer calories are turned into stored fat, and you feel less hungry.

Studies have shown that HCA can suppress fat production by 40 to 80 percent for eight to twelve hours after you eat. HCA can also reduce caloric intake by 10 percent. In a remarkable 1997 study, subjects lost an average of fourteen pounds in two months while supplementing HCA and following a controlled diet. What is remarkable about the study is that the subjects continued to lose weight—another sixteen pounds on average—over the next twelve months of HCA supplementation with no dietary restrictions. Combining HCA with a thermogenic formula (a substance that increases fat burning) creates an even greater effect. According to herbalist Michael Tierra, *Garcinia cambogia* is one of the very safest of herbs and can be used for long periods of time. It is free of unpleasant or dangerous side effects.

Dosage: The usual dosage is 500 mg three times per day. Combine with chromium and a thermogenic formula for best results. Also consume a diet low in harmful fats and high in good fats.

Bitter Orange (*Citrus aurantium*)

Bitter orange works in three ways to aid in weight loss: it stimulates weight loss by enhancing thermogensis (the burning of fat); it builds lean muscle; and it increases physical performance by making fat available for energy. Many experts believe enhancing thermogensis is the most important factor for successful weight loss. Yet some weight-loss products that enhance thermogensis have negative side effects. *Citrus aurantium*, or bitter orange, has been compared to *Ephedra* (another weight-loss supplement). However, unlike *Ephedra* it promotes weight loss without the side effects of nervousness and insomnia. In other words, bitter orange has the benefits of *Ephedra* without the negative central nervous system and cardiovascular side effects.

Research has shown that bitter orange stimulates the receptors that increase the rate at which body stores release fat (lipolysis); bitter orange also increases the metabolic rate (thermogensis), which burns calories. Unlike Ephedra, it minimizes the effect on receptors that have a negative effect on heart rate and blood pressure. It gives the body greater energy, allowing more energy for exercise, and it helps minimize the loss of lean muscle tissue. Bitter orange can also help increase the burning of calories after eating, and it may increase resting metabolic rate, allowing calorie burning when the person is not active. Also unlike *Ephedra*, which can easily cross the blood brain barrier, causing negative nervous system and cardiovascular effects, bitter orange does not cross the blood brain barrier and, therefore, does not have negative side effects.

Dosage: If using the liquid extract, take about ½ tsp (2 mL to 3mL) three times per day. If using the capsules, take one 320-mg capsule (4 percent alkalods) five times per day.

Fiber

Eating fiber is one of the best ways to lose weight. Fiber makes you feel full. It also encourages weight loss by enhancing blood sugar control and insulin effects, by controlling cholesterol, by helping clean the body out and by reducing the amount of calories absorbed by the body.

Fiber is found in plant foods and in supplements, such as psyllium, flaxseeds, guar gum and apple pectin. Most people lose 50 to 100 percent more weight by adding fiber to their diet, rather than by restricting calories.

Dosage: Start by adding as much fiber as you can to your diet. Also, take 10 grams of guar gum before lunch and dinner. For psyllium, flaxseeds and apple pectin, start with 1 to 2 grams before meals and at bedtime, and increase to 5 grams before meals and at bedtime. Some experts believe you need at least 35 grams a day. Drink plenty of water, eight glasses a day, to help the fiber expand. This will make you feel full.

Coenzyme Q10 (CoQ10)

This powerful antioxidant can help you lose weight by getting rid of excess fluid in your body and by increasing energy by feeding the ATP cycle in the body. As many as 50 percent of overweight people are deficient in CoQ10.

Dosage: Take 100 to 400 mg a day. Start slowly and increase as needed.

Dandelion Leaf

Taking dandelion leaf is another excellent way to get rid of excess fluid in the body.

Dosage: Take 40 to 80 drops three times per day on an empty stomach.

Lipotropic Factors (Choline, Methionine, Betaine and Inositol)

The liver is responsible for breaking down fat, and this function is reduced in many people. Lipotropics can help improve this function. They enhance the decongestion of the liver, improving liver function, and they encourage fat metabolism, helping you to lose weight.

Dosage: 1,000 mg a day of lipotropics: combine choline, methionine, betaine and inositol.

Kelp

Kelp is best known for its ability to positively affect an underactive thyroid, a cause of weight gain. The iodine in kelp helps to correct an underactive thyroid and encourages metabolic activity. Iodine assists in making thyroid hormones, which are necessary for maintaining normal metabolism. By supplying many other minerals to the body, kelp provides extra assurance to those on a diet that key nutrients are not missing.

Dosage: Take a kelp-based supplement that contains 1,000 mcg of iodine.

Chastetree Berry

You guessed it—high estrogen levels can actually cause weight gain. The more unnecessary estrogen you have, the harder it can be to lose weight. See Chapter 6 for many great ideas to help lower elevated estrogen levels, and start with this stellar herb for women.

Dosage: Take 3 to 6 grams of the dried and ground berries three times a day. If you are using the tincture, take 30 drops three times a day. Chastetree berry is often standardized for 0.5 percent agnuside. If you are using a standard zed tablet (this form is preferable), take 175 to 225 mg daily; if you are taking a star dardized liquid extract, take ½ tsp (2 mL) a day.

Finally, the End of Excess Weight

With a little time and effort, you will be pleasantly surprised to see how good you feel, how good you look, and how much energy you have. Just don't forget to eat well, and exercise daily to achieve good life habits so you can maintain a healthy weight, a balanced body and good health for life.

The Protocol for Weight Loss

Eat lots of fiber, and cut out empty foods. At the beginning of meals, eat a large salad with flaxseed oil dressing or drink vegetable juice to ensure that you get adequate nutrition and that you don't overeat. Don't skip meals, and do exercise daily. Also try acupuncture: it is fantastic for losing weight and toning the body.

Guar gum: *10 grams of guar gum before lunch and dinner. Start slowly 1 to 2 grams, one time per day, and then build up.*

Alternately:

Flax, pysllium and apple pectin: *1 to 2 grams four times per day on an empty stomach (before meals and at bedtime). Slowly increase to 5 grams before meals and at bedtime. Drink plenty of water (eight glasses a day) to help the fiber expand and make you feel full.*

Chromium: *200 mcg once per day with food for the first week; increase to 400 mcg for the second week. Week three, increase your intake, if needed, to 600 mcg with food. This is best done with a practitioner. Diabetics must monitor their insulin levels.*

This may be all you need to bring your body back into balance. However, if after three months you are not seeing positive results, you may want to consider some additional support. Try one or more of:

Garcinia cambogia (HCA): *500 mg 3 times per day. Combine with chromium and a thermogenic formula for best results. Eat a diet low in bad fats.*

Lipotropic factors: *1,000 mg in total of choline, methionine, betaine and inositol per day.*

continued   137

Bitter orange: *About ½ a teaspoon (2 mL to 3 mL) of the liquid extract three times per day. Or take 320-mg capsules (4 percent alkaloids) five times per day.*

Dandelion root: *40 drops three times per day on an empty stomach.*

Coenzyme Q10: *Take 100 to 400 mg a day. Start slowly and increase as needed.*

Chastetree berry: *Take 3 to 6 grams of the dried and ground berries three times per day. If you are using the tincture, take 30 drops three times per day. Chastetree berry is often standardized for 0.5 percent agnuside. If you are using a standardized tablet (this form is preferable), take 175 to 225 mg daily; if you are taking a standardized liquid extract, take ½ tsp (2 mL) per day.*

If your thyroid is low

Kelp: *Take a kelp-based supplement that contains 1,000 mcg of iodine.*

CONCLUSION

Wrapping It All Up

S o by now you are feeling great about yourself, looking good and feeling healthy. And you did it all yourself. You took control, balanced your hormones, and got rid of unwanted period pain, PMS and all those other nasty, unwanted health conditions that women can have when things are out of balance.

So it is time to share your success with all of your friends. Don't keep it quiet; let them all know what you did to help yourself. Give them the helping hand that you gave yourself. Empower them, as you empowered yourself. Tell your daughters, your mothers, your friends—all the women you know—that they do not have to live in pain and discomfort from unbalanced hormones. Help them to have the most productive, happy, healthy lives they can.

END NOTES

Chapter 2: Understanding PMS

1. Different sources cite slightly different variants of these numbers. See, for example, American College of Obstetrics and Gynecology (ACOG), committee opinion. *Int J Gyn and Obstet* 1995; 50:80 (cited in Hudson T. *Women's Encyclopedia of Natural Medicine*. Los Angeles, CA: Keats Publishing, 1999) and Murray MT. *Premenstrual Syndrome*. Rocklin, CA: Prima Publishing, 1997.

2. Watkins PB, *et al*. Aminotransferase elevations in healthy adults receiving 4 grams of acetaminophen daily: a randomized controlled trial. *JAMA* 2006; 296:87-93.

Chapter 3: The Causes of PMS

1. Murray, Michael T., ND, *Premenstrual Syndrome* (Rocklin, CA: Prima Publishing, 1997), pp. 4-5.

2. Abraham GE. Nutritional factors in the etiology of the premenstrual tension syndromes. *J Reprod Med* 1983; 28:446-64.

3. Chuong CJ, *et al*. Periovulatory betaendorphin levels in premenstrual syndrome. *Obstet Gynecol* 1995; 83:755-60.

4. Barnhart KT, *et al*. A clinician's guide to the premenstrual syndrome. *Med Clin North Am* 1995; 79:1457-72.

5. Bermond P. Therapy of side effects of oral contraceptive agents with B6. *Acta Vitaminol-Enzymol* 1982; 4:45-54.

6. Brayshaw ND, Brayshaw DD. Thyroid hypofunction in premenstrual syndrome. *New Engl J Med* 1986; 315:1486-7.

Chapter 4: The Conventional Approach to PMS

1. Brown, Donald, ND, *et al. Healthnotes Clinical Essentials*, Vol. 1 (Portland, OR: Healthnotes, 2000).

2. Hudson, Tori,ND, *Women's Encyclopedia of Natural Medicine* (Los Angeles, CA: Keats Publishing, 1999), p.74.

3. DeMarco, Carolyn, MD, *Take Charge of Your Body* (Aurora, ON: The Well Women Press, 1995), pp. 46-51.

4. Murray, Michael T., ND, *Natural Alternatives to Over-the-Counter and Prescription Drugs* (New York, NY: William Morrow and Company, 1994), p.223.

5. Brooks PM, Potter SR, Buchanan WW. NSAID and osteoarthritis—help or hindrance. *J Rheumatol* 1982; 9:3-5; Shield MJ. Anti-inflammatory drugs and their

effects on cartilage synthesis and renal function. *Eur J Rheum Inflam* 1993; 13:7-16; Ghosh P. Evaluation of disease progression during nonsteroidal anti-inflammatory drug treatment: experimental models. *Osteoarthritis Cartilage* 1999; 7:340-2; Dingle JT. Cartilage maintenance in osteoarthritis: interaction of cytokines, NSAID and prostaglandins in articular cartilage damage and repair. *J Rheumatol Suppl* 1991; 28:30-37.

6. Balon R, *et al.* Sexual dysfunction during antidepressant treatment. *J Clin Psychiatry* 1993; 54:209-12.

Chapter 5: The Natural Approach to PMS: Dietary Changes

1. Abraham GE. Nutritional factors in the etiology of the premenstrual tension syndromes. *J Reprod Med* 1983; 28:446-64.

2. Goldin BR, *et al.* Estrogen patterns and plasma levels in vegetarian and omnivorous women. *New Engl J Med* 1982; 307:1542-7.

3. Longcope C, *et al.* The effects of a low fat diet on estrogen metabolism. *J Clin Endocrinol Metab* 1987; 64:1246-50.

4. Yudkin J, Eisa O. Dietary sucrose and oestradiol concentration in young men. *Ann Nutr Metabol* 1988; 32:53-5.

5. Rossignol AM, Bonnlander H. Prevalence and severity of the premenstrual syndrome. Effects of foods and beverages that are sweet or high in sugar content. *J Reprod Med* 1991; 36:132-6.

6. *Ibid.*

7. Falck F, *et al.* Pesticides and polychlorinated biphenyl residues in human breast lipids and their relation to breast cancer. *Archives of Environ Health* 1992; 47:143-6.

8. Northrup, Christiane, MD, *Women's Bodies, Women's Wisdom* (Toronto ON: Bantam Books, 1994).

Chapter 6: The Natural Approach to PMS: Herbs and Supplements

1. Loch E-G, *et al.* Treatment of premenstrual syndrome with a phytopharmaceutical formulation containing *Vitex agnus castus. Journal of Women's Health & Gender-Based Medicine* 2000; 9:315-320.

2. Dittmar FW, *et al.* Premenstrual syndrome: Treatment with a phytopharmaceutical. *TW Gynakologie* 1992; 5:60-8.

3. Schellenberg R, Kunze G, Pfaff E, *et al.* Treatment for the premenstrual syndrome with agnus-castus fruit extract: prospective, randomized, placebo controlled study. *BMJ* 2001 Jan; 22; 134-7.

4. Hoffmann, David. *Holistic Herbal* (Shaftesbury, Dorset: Element Books, 1996), p.164.

5. Bohnert KJ. The use of *Vitex agnus castus* for hyperprolactinemia. *Quart Rev Natural Med* 1997; Spring:19-21; Berger D, *et al.*, *Efficacy of Vitex agnus-castus* L. extract Ze440 in patients with pre-menstrual syndrome. *Arch Gynecol Obstet* 2000; 264:150-3; Schellenberg R., Kunze G, Pfaff E, et al., Treatment for the premenstrual syndrome with agnus-castus fruit extract: prospective, randomized, placebo controlled study. *BMJ* 2001 Jan; 322:134-7.

6. Mowrey, Daniel, Ph.D, *Herbal Tonic Therapies* (New Canaan, CT: Keats Publishing, 1993), p.7.

7. Liske E. Physiological investigation of a unique extract of black cohosh (*Cimecifugae racemosae rhizome*): a 6-month clinical study demonstrates no systemic estrogenic effect. *Journal of Women's Health & Gender Based Medicine* 2002; 11(2):163-74; *Menopause* 1998. See also Steven Foster. Black Cohosh: A Literature Review. *Herbalgram* #45.

8. Schildge E. Essay on the treatment of premenstrual and menopausal mood swings and depressive states. *Rigelh Biol Umsch* 1964; 19(2):18-22.

9. Wyatt KM, *et al.*, Efficacy of vitamin B6 in the treatment of premenstrual syndrome: systematic review. *BMJ* 1999; 318:1375-81.

10. Barr W. Pyridoxine supplements in the premenstrual syndrome. *Practitioner* 1984; 228:425-7.

11. Abraham. GE. Nutritional factors in the etiology of the premenstrual tension syndromes. *J Reprod Med* 1983; 28:446-64; Piesse JW. Nutritional factors in the premenstrual syndrome. *Int Clin Nutr Rev* 1984; 4:54-81.

12. Abraham, GE. Nutritional factors in the etiology of the premenstrual tension syndromes. *J Repro Med* 1983;28: 446-64.

13. Thys-Jacobs, *et al.* Calcium carbonate and the premenstrual syndrome: effects on premenstrual and menstrual symptoms. *Am J Obstet Gynecol* 1998; 179:444-52.

14. Bertone-Johnson ER, *et al,* Calcium and vitamin D intake and risk of incident premenstrual syndrome. *Arch Intern Med* 2005; 165:1246-1252.

15. London RS, *et al*. The effect of alpha-tocopherol on premenstrual symptomatology: a double-blind study. II: endocrine correlates. *J Am Coll Nutr* 1984; 3:351-6.

16. Gaby, Alan R., MD, *Preventing and Reversing Osteoporosis* (Rocklin, CA: Prima Publishing, 1994), p.55.

17. Erasmus U, *Fats That Heal, Fats That Kill* (Burnaby. BC: Alive Books, 1995).

18. Murray, Michael T., ND, *5-HTP* (New York, NY: Bantam Books, 1998), p.224.

19. Maurizio F, *et al*. A Double-blind, randomized trial of St John's wort, fluoxetine, and placebo in major depressive disorder. *J Clin Psychopharmacol* 2005; 25:441-447.

20. Akhondzadeh S, *et al*. Passionflower in the treatment of generalized anxiety: a pilot double-blind randomized controlled trial with oxazepam. *J Clin Pharm Ther* 2001; 26:363-7.

21. Zeigler G, *et al*. Efficacy and tolerability of valerian extract LI 156 compared with oxazepam in the treatment of non-organic insomnia—a randomized, double-blind, comparative clinical study. *Eur J Med Res* 2002; 25; 7:480-6.

22. Chakmakjian Z, *et al*. The effects of a nutritional supplement, Optivate for women, on premenstrual tension syndrome: effect of symptomatology, using a double-blind crossover design. *J Appl Nutr* 1985; 37:12.

Chapter 7: Dysmenorrhea (Painful Periods)

1. Penland J, Johnson P. Dietary calcium and manganese effects on menstrual cycle symptoms. *Am J Obstet Gynecol* 1993; 168:1417-23.

2. Northrup, Christiane, MD, *Women's Bodies, Women's Wisdom* (New York, NY: Bantam Books, 1995), p.115.

3. Hudgins A. Niacin for dysmenorrhea. *Am Prac Digest Trea* 1952; 3: 892-3.

4. Hudgins A. Vitamins P, C and niacin for dysmenorrhea therapy. *West J Surg Gynecol* 1954; 62: 610-11.

5. Butler E, McKnight E. Vitamin E in the treatment of primary dysmenorrhea. *Lancet* 1955; 1:844-7.

6. Ziaei S, *et al*., A randomized placebo-controlled trial to determine the effect of vitamin E in treatment of primary dysmenorrhoea. *Br J Obstet Gynaecol* 2001; 108:1181-3.

7. Ziaei S, *et al*., A randomized controlled trial of vitamin E in the treatment of primary dysmenorrhoea. *Br J Obstet Gynaecol* 2005; 112:466-9.

Chapter 8: Menorrhagia (Excessive Blood Flow)

1. Cohen JD, Rubin HW. Functional menorrhagia: treatment with bioflavonoids and vitamin C. *Curr Ther Res* 1960; 2:539-42.

Chapter 9: Amenorrhea (Absence of Periods)

1. Crawford, Amanda McQuade. *Herbal Remedies for Women* (Rocklin, CA: Prima, 1997); Hobbs, Christopher, *Vitex: The Women's Herb* (Santa Cruz, CA: Botanica Press, 1996).

2. DeMarco, Carolyn, MD, *Take Charge of Your Body* (Aurora, ON: The Well Women Press, 1995), p.151.

3. *Ibid.*, p.239

4. Milewica A, *et al. Vitex agnus castus* extract in the treatment of luteal phase defects due to hyperprolactinemia. Results of a randomized placebo-controlled double-blind study. *Arzneim-Forsch Drug Res* 1993; 43:752-6.

5. Bove, Mary, ND, Costarella, Linda, ND, *Herbs for Women's Health* (New Canaan, CT: Keats Publishing, 1997), p.20.

6. Hudson, Tori, ND, *Women's Encyclopedia of Natural Medicine* (Los Angeles, CA: Keats Publishing, 1999), p. 20.

7. Ohta H, *et al.* Effects of 1-year ipriflavone treatment on lumbar bone mineral density and bone metabolic markers in postmenopausal women with low bone mass. *Horm Res* 1999; 51:178-83; Agnusdei D, *et al.* A double-blind, placebo-controlled trial of ipriflavone for prevention of postmenopausal spinal bone loss. *Calcif Tissue Int* 1997; 61: 142-7. There are at least five other studies.

Chapter 10: Preventing and Treating Fibrocystic Breast Disease

1. Minton JP, *et al.* Clinical and biochemical studies on methylxanthine-related fibrocystic breast disease. *Surgery* 1981; 90:229-304.

2. Pye JK, Mansel RE, Hughes LE. Clinical experience of drug treatments for mastalgia. *Lancet* 1985; ii:373–7; Harding C, *et al.* Hormone replacement therapy-induced mastalgia responds to evening primrose oil. *Br J Surg* 1996; 83(Suppl 1):24; Preece PE, *et al.* Evening primrose oil (EFAMOL) for mastalgia. In: *Clinical Uses of Essential Fatty Acids*, ed. DF Horrobin, (Montreal: Eden Press), 1982, 147–54; Pashby N, *et al.* A clinical trial of evening primrose oil in mastalgia. *Br J Surg* 1981; 68:801-24.

Chapter 11: Eliminating Ovarian Cysts and Uterine Fibroids

1. Adlercreutz H, *et al*. Dietary phytoestrogens and cancer: *in vitro* and *in vivo* studies. *J Steroid Biochem Molec Biol* 1992; 41:331-7.

2. Braden A, Hart N, Lamberton J. The oestrogenic activity and metabolism of certain isoflavones in sheep. *Aust J of Agr Res* 1967; 18:335-48.

Chapter 12: Help for Endometriosis

1. Gladstar, Rosemary, *Herbal Healing for Women* (New York NY: Fireside, 1993).

Chapter 13: Safe Help for Pregnancy

1. Vutyavanich T, *et al*. Ginger for nausea and vomiting in pregnancy: randomized, double-masked, placebo-controlled trial. *Obstet Gynecol* 2001; 97(4):577-82; Keating A, Chez R. Ginger syrup as an antiemetic in early pregnancy. *Alternative Therapies*. 2002; 8(5):89-91.

2. Fischer-Rasmussen W, *et al*. Ginger treatment of hyperemisis graridarum. *Eur J Obstet Gynecol Reprod Biol* 38, 19-24, 1990.

3. Bergner P. Is ginger safe during pregnancy? *Medical Herbalism* 1991; 3(3):7.

4. Fulder and Tenne. Ginger as an Anti-nausea Remedy in Pregnancy: The Issue of Safety, *Herbalgram* #38, 1996.

5. Tierra, Michael, L.Ac., O.M.D., *The Way of Herbs* (New York, NY: Pocket Books, 1998).

6. Hojo M, August P. Calcium metabolism in normal and hypertensive pregnancy. *Semin Nephrol* 1995; 15:504–11 [review].

7. DerSimonian R, Levine RJ. Resolving discrepancies between a meta-analysis and a subsequent large controlled trial. *JAMA* 1999;282:664–70 [review]; Ritchie LD, King JC. Dietary calcium and pregnancy-induced hypertension: is there a relation? *Am J Clin Nutr* 2000;71(5 Suppl):1371–4S [review]; Villar J, Belizan JM. Same nutrient, different hypotheses: disparities in trials of calcium supplementation during pregnancy. *Am J Clin Nutr* 2000;71(5 Suppl):1375–9S [review].

8. Altra BM, *et al*. Magnesium deficiency-induced spasm of umbilical vessels: Relation to preeclempsia, hypertension, growth retardation. *Science* 1983;221:376-8; Spatling L, Spatling G. Magnesium supplementation in pregnancy. A double-blind study. *Br J Obstet Gynaecol* 1988;95:120-5; Rudnicki M,

et al. The effect of magnesium on maternal blood pressure in pregnancy-induced hypertension. A randomized double-blind placebo-controlled trial. *Acta Obstet Gynecol Scand* 1991; 70:445-50.

9. Tabacova S, Balabaeva L, Little RE. Maternal exposure to exogenous nitrogen compounds and complications of pregnancy. *Arch Environ Health* 1997; 52:341–7; Mutlu-Turkoglu U, Ademoglu E, Ibrahimoglu L, *et al.* Imbalance between lipid peroxidation and antioxidant status in preeclampsia. *Gynecol Obstet Invest* 1998;46:37–40; Mikhail MS, *et al.* Preeclempsia and antioxidant nutrients: Decreased plasma levels of reduced ascorbic acid, alpha-tocopherol, and beta-carotene in women with preeclempsia. *Am J Obstet Gynecol* 1994; 171:150-7.

10. Chappell LC, *et al.* Effect of antioxidants on the occurrence of pre-eclampsia in women at increased risk: a randomised trial. *Lancet* 1999; 354:810–6.

Chapter 14: How to Have a Healthy, Happy Menopause

1. Nestel PJ, *et al.* Isoflavones from red clover improve systemic arterial compliance but not plasma lipids in menopausal women. *J Clin Endocrinol Metab* 1999; 84:895–8

2. Stolze H. An alternative to treat menopausal complaints. *Gynecology* 1982;1:14-6; Warnecke G. Influencing menopausal symptoms with a phytotherapeutic agent. Successful therapy with *Cimicifuga* mono-extract. *Med Welt* 1985;36(2):871-4; Stoll W. Phytopharmacon influences atrophic vaginal epithelium: double-blind study—*Cimicifuga* vs. estrogenic substances. *Therapeutikon* 1987; 1:23-31.

3. Stoll W. Phytopharmacon influences atrophic vaginal epithelium: double-blind study—*Cimicifuga* vs. estrogenic substances. *Therapeutikon* 1987;1:23-31; Duker E, *et al.* Effects of extracts from *Cimicifuga* racemosa on gonadotropin release in menopausal women and ovariectomized rats. *Planta Med* 1991; 57:420-4.

4. Stolze H. An alternative to treat menopausal complaints. *Gynecology* 1982;1:14-6; Warnecke G. Influencing menopausal symptoms with a phytotherapeutic agent. Successful therapy with *Cimicifuga* mono-extract. *Med Welt* 1985;36(2):871-4; Stoll W. Phytopharmacon influences atrophic vaginal epithelium: double-blind study—*Cimicifuga* vs. estrogenic substances. *Therapeutikon* 1987; 1:23-31.

5. Wuttke W, Seidlova-Wuttke D, Gorkow C. The *Cimicifuga* preparation BNO 1055 vs conjugated estrogens in a double-blind placebo-controlled study: effects on menopause symptoms and bone markers. *Maturitas* 2003:44 Suppl 1; 67-77.

6. Nesselhut T, *et al.* Studies of the proliferative potency of phytodrugs with estrogen-like effect in breast cancer cells. *Arch Gynecol Obstet* 1993;817-8; Hostanska K, *et al. Cimicifuga racemosa* extract inhibits proliferation of estrogen receptor-positive and negative human breast carcinoma cell lines by induction of apoptosis. *Breast Cancer Res Treat.* March 2004; 84:151-160.

7. Christy CJ. Vitamin E in menopause. *Am J Ob Gyn* 1945;50:84-7 Mclaren HC. Vitamin E in the menopause. *Br Med J* 1949;ii:1378-81; Finkler RS. The effect of vitamin E in the menopause. *J Clin Endocrinol Metab* 1949; 9:89-94.

8. Smith CJ. Non-hormonal control of vasomotor flushing in menopausal patients. Chic Med 1964; 67:193-5.

Chapter 15: Prevention and Treatment of Osteoporosis

1. Feskanich D, *et al.* Milk, dietary calcium, and bone fractures in women: a 12-year prospective study. *Am J Public Health* 1997; 87:992-7.

Chapter 16: Healthy Weight Loss

1. McCarthy MF. Hypothesis: Sensitization of insulin-dependent hypothalamic glucoreceptors may account for the fat-reducing effects of chromium picolinate. *J Optimal Nutr* 1993;21:36-53.

2. Murray, Michael T., ND, *Natural Alternatives for Weight Loss* (New York: William Morrow and Company, 1996).

3. Evans GW, Pouchnik DJ. Composition and biological activity of chromium-pyridine carbosylate complexes. *J Inorganic Biochemistr* 1993; 49:177-87.

BIBLIOGRAPHY

Blumenthal, Mark, *et al*, eds. *The Complete German Commission E Monographs*. Austin, TX: American Botanical Council, 1998.

Blumenthal, Mark, ed. *Herbalgram* #42. Austin, TX: American Botanical Council, 1998.

—. *Herbalgram* #45. Austin, TX: American Botanical Council, 1999.

Bove, Mary, ND and Linda Costarella, ND. *Herbs for Women's Health*. New Canaan, CT: Keats Publishing, 1997.

Brown, Donald J, ND, *et al. Clinical Essentials*. Portland, OR: Healthnotes, 2000.

Brown, Donald J, ND, ed. *Healthnotes* Vol.7, No.1. Portland, OR: Healthnotes, 2000

Crawford, Amanda McQuade, MNIMH. *Herbal Remedies for Women*. Rocklin, CA: Prima Publishing, 1997.

DeMarco, Carolyn, MD. *Take Charge of Your Body*. Aurora, ON: The Well Women Press, 1995.

Erasmus, Udo, Ph.D. *Fats that Heal; Fats that Kill*. Burnaby, BC: Alive Books, 1997.

Gaby, Alan R, MD. *Preventing and Reversing Osteoporosis*. Rocklin, CA: Prima Publishing, 1994.

Gladstar, Rosemary. *Herbal Healing for Women*. New York, NY: Fireside, 1993.

Gursche, Siegfried, MH, ed. *Encyclopedia of Natural Healing*. Burnaby, BC: Alive Books, 1997.

Hobbs, Christopher, L.Ac. *Vitex: The Women's Herb*. Santa Cruz, CA: Botanica Press, 1996.

Hoffmann, David, MNIMH. *Holistic Herbal.* Shaftesbury, Dorset: Element Books, 1996.

Hudson, Tori, ND. *Women's Encyclopedia of Natural Medicine.* Los Angeles, CA: Keats Publishing, 1999.

Jacob, Stanley W, MD, *et al. The Miracle of MSM.* New York, NY: G.P. Putnam's Sons, 1999.

Lee, John, R, MD. *What Your Doctor May* Not *Tell You About Menopause.* New York, NY: Warner Books, 1996.

Love, Susan M, MD and Karen Lindsey. *Dr. Susan Love's Breast Book.* Reading, MS: Perseus Books, 1995.

Mindell, Earl, R.Ph., Ph.D. *Earl Mindell's Supplement Bible.* New York, NY: Firseside, 1998.

Mowrey, Daniel B, Ph.D. *Herbal Tonic Therapies.* New Canaan, CT: Keats Publishing, 1993.

Murray, Michael T, ND and Joseph Pizzorno, ND. *Encyclopedia of Natural Medicine,* 2nd Edition. Rocklin, CA: Prima Publishing, 1998.

Murray, Michael T, ND. *Premenstrual Syndrome.* Rocklin, CA: Prima Publishing, 1997.

—. *Natural Alternatives to Prozac.* New York, NY: William Morrow and Company, 1996.

—. *Natural Alternatives to Over-the-Counter and Prescription Drugs.* New York, NT: William Morrow and Company, 1994.

—. *5-HTP.* New York, NY: Bantam Books, 1998.

—. *The Healing Power of Herbs,* 2nd Edition. Rocklin, CA: Prima Publishing, 1995.

—. *Encyclopedia of Nutritional Supplements.* Rocklin, CA: Prima Publishing, 1996.

Northrup, Christiane, MD. *Women's Bodies, Women's Wisdom.* New York, NY: Bantam Books, 1994.

Pizzorno, Joseph E, Jr, ND and Michael T Murray, ND, eds. *Textbook of Natural Medicine,* 2nd Edition. London: Churchill Livingstone, 1999.

Tierra, Michael, L.Ac., OMD. *The Way of Herbs,* 2nd Edition. New York, NY: Pocket Books, 1998.

INDEX